Praise for
METABOLIC FREEDOM

"*Metabolic Freedom* cuts through the noise of modern health myths and offers a refreshing perspective on fat loss, focusing on root causes rather than symptoms. Ben's deep understanding of metabolism and practical tools like the 30-day reset make this an indispensable guide for anyone seeking lasting health and vitality."

— **Dr. Jason Fung**, *New York Times* best-selling author of *The Obesity Code*

"*Metabolic Freedom* is a transformative journey toward vibrant health and metabolic balance. Blending personal experience with science-backed strategies, Ben Azadi offers practical tools to heal your metabolism, balance hormones, and break free from the cycle of diets and chronic health struggles. Complete with a 30-day reset plan, this book is an essential guide for anyone seeking lasting wellness and vitality."

— **Robert Lufkin, M.D.**, *New York Times* best-selling author of
Lies I Taught in Medical School and medical school professor

"Ben Azadi's *Metabolic Freedom* is a game-changer for anyone ready to break free from the cycle of yo-yo dieting and metabolic dysfunction. Ben masterfully combines ancient healing tools including keto and fasting with cutting-edge biohacks to help you unlock your body's innate intelligence. From understanding the root causes of metabolic issues to implementing his 30-Day Metabolic Freedom Reset, this book provides a practical, science-backed road map to lasting health and vitality. If you're ready to transform your metabolism and reclaim your energy, this is the guide you've been waiting for."

— **JJ Virgin**, 4x *New York Times* best-selling author

"*Metabolic Freedom* by Ben Azadi is more than just a book—it's a wake-up call for anyone stuck in metabolic dysfunction. It simplifies complex health strategies like keto, fasting, and biohacking into actionable steps you can start today."

— **Dr. Eric Berg**, human biologist and biohacker

"At last, a book on metabolism that uncovers the true root causes of energy loss, brain fog, unexplained weight gain, and even diabetes. *Metabolic Freedom* breaks free from the conventional diet-focused approach that often leaves people feeling stuck and disappointed by limited or nonexistent results. This isn't just another diet book—it's a transformative guide to understanding and revitalizing your metabolism like never before."

— **Dr. Daniel Pompa**, author of *Beyond Fasting* and founder of Pompa Program

"With *Metabolic Freedom*, Ben Azadi delivers an impactful, empowering blueprint for unlocking your body's innate healing potential. Packed with insights on intermittent fasting, ketogenic diets, and biohacking, this book equips you to overcome metabolic dysfunction and live your healthiest life. It's not just a book—it's a lifeline for anyone ready to take control of their health. Highly recommended reading for not only my patients but clients as well!"

— **Cynthia Thurlow, NP**, women's health expert, author, and podcast host of *Everyday Wellness*

"*Metabolic Freedom*—what a beautiful, high-concept title! We all deserve to be free from the health hazards of heavily processed modern food, and even ill-advised conventional approaches to weight loss. As someone who helped popularize the concept of 'metabolic flexibility,' I can confirm that Ben's new book is a fantastic resource for anyone wishing to improve their metabolic health, lose excess body fat the right way (and keep it off forever with minimal effort), and prevent disease."

— **Mark Sisson**, ancestral health movement founding father and *New York Times* best-selling author of *The Primal Blueprint*, *The Keto Reset Diet*, and *Born to Walk*

"What Ben Azadi does in *Metabolic Freedom* is open your eyes to food propaganda, educate you about what real food is, and protect your future self from falling for the slick ads of big-food companies."

— **Ken D. Berry, M.D.**, author of *Lies My Doctor Told Me*

"Every cell in your body is a miracle of biotechnology. Ben Azadi has given us a clear path to restoring their metabolism at the cellular level. Read this book and learn from one of the best."

— **Cate Shanahan, M.D.**, *New York Times* best-selling author

"Ben Azadi has cracked the code to metabolic health! *Metabolic Freedom* isn't just another book—it's a game-changer. This is about getting to the root cause, not masking symptoms. Ben breaks down the science into simple, actionable steps so you can take control of your energy, burn fat like a machine, and finally feel *alive* again. If you're ready to unlock your body's innate intelligence, fire on all cylinders, and crush life every single day, *Metabolic Freedom* is the blueprint you've been waiting for."

— **Gary Brecka**, human biologist and biohacker

"In *Metabolic Freedom*, author Ben Azadi provides a road map to reclaiming your metabolic health in a world plagued by misinformation, disinformation, and misleading marketing. With science-backed strategies shared in easily accessible plain language along with personal anecdotes and actionable steps, Ben Azadi provides key strategies for achieving sustainable weight loss, balanced hormones, and youthful energy."

— **Dr. William Davis**, author of #1 *New York Times* bestseller, *Wheat Belly*

"Metabolic freedom is the promised land of health, healing, and thriving with great energy, mental clarity, fat burning, strength and resilience to handle the challenges of life. Unfortunately, in our society today, very few people experience this desired physiological state. Ben Azadi has written an authoritative guide on how you can flip the metabolic switch and get freedom in your health! I highly recommend this book!"

— **Dr. David Jockers, DNM, DC, MS**, author of *The Keto Metabolic Breakthrough* and *The Fasting Transformation*

"Ben Azadi has a beautiful way of simplifying complex health concepts, making them accessible and actionable for everyone. In his 30-day guide to mastering your metabolism, he shatters the broken mindset we've been taught about health and empowers you with the knowledge to completely transform your body from the inside out. Prepare to be blown away by how quickly you—and your cells— can start fresh with Ben's easy, realistic plan that fits seamlessly into your life. With over a million inspired followers and counting, Ben isn't just teaching these principles—he's living proof that they work. This book is your road map to lasting health and vitality, guided by someone who has truly walked the walk."

— **Dr. Melissa Sonners**, host of *Be Inspired Mama* podcast and Hay House author

"Ben Azadi has written a must-read for anyone looking to restore their metabolism and regain control of their health. He provides readers with a masterclass in understanding the root cause of disease as well as a 30-day reset to achieve metabolic freedom. This book is packed with insights that will change your life."

— **Megan Ramos**, *New York Times* best-selling author of *Life in the Fasting Lane* and co-founder of The Fasting Method

"*Metabolic Freedom* gives readers a road map for personalizing their metabolism and making it work to achieve better health."

— **William W. Li, M.D.**, *New York Times* best-selling author of *Eat to Beat Disease*, president and medical director, the Angiogenesis Foundation

"In *Metabolic Freedom*, Ben Azadi provides an empowering guide to reclaiming your health through the transformative power of keto, fasting, and detox strategies. This book is a must-read for women looking to support their hormones, optimize energy, and break free from the cycle of metabolic chaos. It's not just about weight loss—it's about achieving true vitality and thriving at every stage of life."

— **Carrie Jones, ND, FABNE, MPH, MSCP**

METABOLIC
FREEDOM

Hay House Titles of Related Interest

YOU CAN HEAL YOUR LIFE, the movie,
starring Louise Hay & Friends
(available as an online streaming video)
www.hayhouse.com/louise-movie

THE SHIFT, the movie,
starring Dr. Wayne W. Dyer
(available as an online streaming video)
www.hayhouse.com/the-shift-movie

***

FAST LIKE A GIRL: A Woman's Guide to Using the Healing Power of Fasting to Burn Fat, Boost Energy, and Balance Hormones, by Dr. Mindy Pelz

REAL SUPERFOODS: Everyday Ingredients to Elevate Your Health, by Ocean Robbins

MEDICAL MEDIUM CLEANSE TO HEAL: Healing Plans for Sufferers of Anxiety, Depression, Acne, Eczema, Lyme, Gut Problems, Brain Fog, Weight Issues, Migraines, Bloating, Vertigo, Psoriasis, Cysts, Fatigue, PCOS, Fibroids, UTI, Endometriosis & Autoimmune, by Anthony William

COMPLETE KETO: A Guide to Transforming Your Body and Your Mind for Life, by Drew Manning

METABOLIC FREEDOM

A 30-DAY GUIDE TO RESTORE YOUR METABOLISM, HEAL HORMONES & BURN FAT

BEN AZADI

HAY HOUSE LLC
Carlsbad, California • New York City
London • Sydney • New Delhi

Published in the United States by: Hay House LLC, www.hayhouse.com®
P.O. Box 5100, Carlsbad, CA, 92018-5100

Project editor: Sally Mason-Swaab • *Indexer:* J S Editorial, LLC
Cover design: Jason Gabbert • *Interior design:* Nick C. Welch • *Interior images:* Courtesy of Ben Azadi

Cataloging-in-Publication Data is on file at the Library of Congress

Hardcover ISBN: 978-1-4019-9436-5
E-book ISBN: 978-1-4019-9437-2
Audiobook ISBN: 978-1-4019-9438-9

10 9 8 7 6 5 4 3 2
1st edition, May 2025

Printed in the United States of America

This product uses responsibly sourced papers, including recycled materials and materials from other controlled sources.

The authorized representative in the EU for product safety and compliance is Penguin Random House Ireland, Morrison Chambers, 32 Nassau Street, Dublin D02 YH68, Ireland. https://eu-contact.penguin.ie

For Cyrus Azadi
Born 1933, died in 2014 from a stroke (a preventable
metabolic condition caused by the complications of his diabetes)

CONTENTS

FOREWORD

Metabolic health is the most important wellness conversation of our time. Every single chronic disease has its roots in poor metabolic health. The growing mental health challenges are exacerbated by an overloaded metabolic system. Even the world's immune system has been compromised by a metabolic system gone awry. As a culture we are in one metabolic mess.

Unfortunately for most people, poor metabolic health has now become the norm, not the exception. As of 2022, 93 percent of Americans are metabolically unhealthy and approximately 2.5 billion adults worldwide have been classified as overweight, with over 890 million of them living with obesity. This means that 43 percent of adults aged 18 years and over are overweight, and 16 percent are obese. And this isn't just an American challenge; it's affecting millions across the globe. According to the World Health Organization; the worldwide prevalence of obesity more than doubled between 1990 and 2022, and if current trends continue, it's predicted that more than half of the global population—over 4 billion people—will be living with overweight or obesity by 2035. The financial impact of this alone is staggering. It is estimated that the global economic impact of overweight and obesity is estimated to reach $4.32 trillion annually by 2035, accounting for nearly 3 percent of the global GDP. This madness needs to stop!

Here's the challenge: changing the direction of your metabolic health is not as easy as it used to be. Our food system has intentionally added harmful ingredients to our foods that have hijacked our taste buds, making us more addicted to toxic ingredients than ever before. Chemicals that are classified as obesogens—ingredients that disrupt the body's hormonal systems, promoting weight gain and fat storage. Chemicals that interfere with our metabolism, appetite regulation, and fat cell development, contributing to this global rise in obesity rates. Perhaps the most harmful part of these chemicals is that you practically need a Ph.D. in biochemistry to interpret them on a nutrition label. Mix a high dose of obesogens with the increasing stress loads, lack of movement, and growing number of toxins that are pouring into our environment, and we have a serious health crisis on our hands.

It's time for a metabolic hero to emerge. Someone who can help us make sense of all of this. Someone who is courageous and patient enough to give us a map that guides us back to metabolic freedom. Enter Ben Azadi, a fierce leader in the health space, whose commitment to helping the world turn its metabolic health around is unwavering. I have known Ben for over ten years now. We have sat together in endless wellness conferences, debated health concepts with other practitioners in brilliant masterminds, and spent endless hours discussing how to motivate people back to health. I know his heart. I have witnessed his unrelenting commitment to serving humanity. I have seen him in action as he has tirelessly helped his community. He is a gift to the metabolic conversation!

Metabolic Freedom is more than a guide—it's a lifeline. In this book, Ben masterfully combines decades of research, personal experience, and practical tools to tackle a problem we all face: a broken relationship with food, hormones, and metabolic health. This book doesn't just promise quick fixes. Instead, it's a deep dive into restoring the innate intelligence of the body—a philosophy I deeply resonate with. Just as I teach my community about the power of fasting, metabolic flexibility, and hormone balance, Ben emphasizes the importance of resetting the metabolism from the ground up.

Perhaps what struck me most about *Metabolic Freedom* is its ability to balance cutting-edge science with actionable steps. Ben simplifies complex topics like autophagy, mitochondrial health, and cellular inflammation into digestible (and inspiring) lessons, helping you take back control of your health. His journey from metabolic dysfunction to vibrant health is a testament to the body's ability to heal itself when given the right tools and environment.

For women, particularly those navigating hormonal shifts like menopause, this book is a treasure trove. Ben's insights on liver health, hormonal regulation, and the role of key nutrients align beautifully with the principles I teach about fasting and resetting hormones. Whether you're dealing with insulin resistance, inflammation, or simply feeling stuck in a cycle of low energy, the solutions offered here—like the 30-Day Metabolic Freedom Reset—are designed to work in harmony with your biology, not against it.

To all readers, I encourage you to approach this book not just as a manual but as a movement. Embrace the ancient healing strategies, biohacks, and nutritional wisdom Ben outlines. Your body is designed to thrive, and with the knowledge in these pages, you can unlock a level of health you may have thought was out of reach.

This isn't just about losing weight or fixing symptoms—it's about reclaiming your life. I'm honored to write this foreword for *Metabolic Freedom* and to champion a book that will undoubtedly empower millions to heal their bodies, restore their vitality, and achieve true metabolic health.

Here's to your journey of transformation and freedom. I know Ben and I are both cheering you on!

— **Dr. Mindy Pelz**
New York Times best-selling author of *Eat Like a Girl,*
Fast Like a Girl, and *The Menopause Reset*

INTRODUCTION

When people decide to take on the formidable task of climbing Mount Everest, they're often assigned a personal sherpa to guide them on their journey. It's common for climbers to experience symptoms of altitude sickness as they trek their way up the mountain. These symptoms begin as subtle annoyances, such as heavy breathing and body aches, until they manifest into serious problems like frostbite and then death. Without a sherpa to guide them, these climbers would likely wind up in the danger zone. Once they're in the danger zone, things get tricky: Most climbers find themselves hopeless and stuck, eventually dying from the severe conditions.

Having been in the health and wellness space since 2008, I've seen many people who are in the metabolic health danger zone . . . and they have no idea. Symptoms are the first signs of trouble, but most people reach for medications or fad diets to cover them up while continuing to step closer to the danger zone.

My goal with this book is to be your sherpa on the journey to health and metabolic freedom. I've created the exact game plan you need to pull yourself out of the danger zone and into the thrive zone.

My (Once) Broken Metabolism

When your metabolism falls apart, every aspect of your life comes crashing down. I know—I've been there. For most of my childhood and early adulthood, I struggled with a broken metabolism. At age 24, when many people are starting their careers or building a family, I was struggling to find the energy to complete simple tasks. The 80 pounds of extra weight I was carrying due to a broken metabolism caused knee pain, lower back pain, autoimmune disease, prediabetes, depression, chronic fatigue, and inflammation. My family physician warned me that my blood sugar kept creeping up within the prediabetes range, and my blood pressure had increased. When I asked him for advice, he simply said, "You need to lose some extra weight. Just eat less and move more." I tried this approach, as many do, only to find myself in worse shape.

1

I remember having several doctors' appointments during which I was told that most of my bloodwork was "normal," yet I felt anything but. The doctors thought I was crazy, but I knew something was interfering with my body. Conversation after conversation only led to more frustration—several prescriptions to aid my symptoms were suggested, but there was not one discussion about the root cause of why I felt and looked inflamed. Like millions of other people, I left each doctor's appointment feeling more discouraged than ever before. I was so hopeless that I began to entertain suicidal thoughts. The only thing that prevented me from taking my life was my mother. Every time I entertained a suicidal thought, I thought about the pain and suffering she would endure.

In the depths of darkness, I also knew deep down that there had to be a way to overcome the uncomfortable symptoms and inflammation I was experiencing. I discovered that there's a blessing in hitting rock bottom: You can use it as a spring-board to discover how magnificent your human body is. You can take all your pain and turn it into purpose.

I was desperate for answers, so I began reading books. I started with books from Dr. Wayne Dyer, who helped me break out of a victim mindset. At the time I was blaming my enabling family members, bad genes, and slow metabolism for my health issues. Dr. Dyer taught me how to take ownership and responsibility for the first time in my life. He said, "Responsibility is your ability to respond to life." Up until that point my ability to respond to life was poor, and then I heard Dr. Dyer say, "If other people are the cause of your problems, you'd have to hire a psychiatrist for the rest of the world, in order for you to get better." After taking responsibility, I immediately stopped being the victim of my history and instead became the victor of my destiny.

How I Achieved Metabolic Health

I made small changes to the food I was fueling my body with, then began to move my body. I had the mindset of one tweak a week. I started digging into research articles and books on metabolism, and I discovered that not all foods are created equal. There are foods that support a healthy metabolism and foods that destroy it. I had been eating foods that were marketed as healthy, but they were actually destroying my body at the cellular level. These were popular health foods, such as whole grains, oatmeal, cereal, canola oil, and many others. These foods were given a stamp of approval by the FDA, the U.S. Department of Agriculture's MyPlate guidelines, and other organizations like the American Diabetes Association and American Heart Association.

After switching to metabolism-supporting foods, such as eggs, meat, butter, and non-starchy vegetables, within just a few days, I felt the shift in my body that I'd been desiring: more mental clarity, fewer suicidal thoughts, and less inflammation; and the weight began to peel off like a snake shedding its excess skin. I knew that if I was going to get well and achieve metabolic health, I needed to find a more unconventional path. I didn't want to rely on medication or extreme diets to mask symptoms. I was determined to find a path that would heal my metabolism for good. This led me to the greatest health tool we have: ancient healing strategies.

When I began to study these principles that have stood the test of time, I knew I was on to something really profound. As Dr. Dyer said, "When you change the way you look at things, the things you look at change." I looked at metabolic health through a different lens, and this moment changed the trajectory of my life in an instant.

Once I discovered the secrets to a healthy, flexible metabolism, I was able to shed over 80 pounds of excess fat—and keep it off for good. I went from 34 percent body fat to 6 percent body fat, from a size 38 waist to a size 30. My energy levels skyrocketed, and the chronic fatigue and pain disappeared. Having a physical six-pack can be great, but more important, I achieved a mental six-pack. Gone were the days of calorie counting, hopelessness, and yo-yo dieting. I achieved something we all desire: true metabolic health.

I've been metabolically healthy and lean ever since I incorporated these ancient healing practices into my life. How was my body able to respond so well to these changes? Am I an outlier? No. What I discovered is that *the human body is built to be self-healing.*

Cracking the Metabolic Code to Health

Inside your body you have the world's greatest physician: innate intelligence. For years I had been blocking my innate intelligence by eating the wrong foods. Once I removed the interference, my body went to work to heal itself. Out of this process, I cracked the metabolic code to health. It doesn't matter what your age is or how many symptoms you are experiencing right now; when you have the combination to the code, you can unlock it.

I became fascinated by the lack of education most people receive about how their metabolism works. I studied and tested the most popular diets and methods for weight loss and have spent the last 17 years working with the most difficult health cases, helping those patients discover which foods support a healthy metabolism and which foods wreck it.

Since 2008, I have taught these metabolic secrets to millions of people across the world. Every single function inside your body is dependent on metabolism, which comes from the Greek *metabole*, meaning to change or transform. Your metabolism takes different substances, such as protein, carbohydrates, fats, body fat, sunshine, and oxygen, and transforms them into energy. When this happens the way your body intended, your metabolism produces energy, buffers oxidative stress (what leads to cell damage), and burns excess fat.

The Sickening Health Statistics

There's never been a more important time to become metabolically healthy. Decade after decade, chronic conditions like cancer, diabetes, autoimmunity, cardiovascular disease, Alzheimer's, hormone imbalance, mental illness, and even chronic fatigue and pain have risen to levels we've never seen before. Many people feel overwhelmed and disheartened by the traditional way of treating these conditions, which usually involves a cookie-cutter approach that masks the symptoms but rarely gets to the cause.

As the Centers for Disease Control and Prevention (CDC) reported, in 2017–2018 the prevalence of obesity among U.S. adults was a whopping 42.4 percent.[1] Another 32.5 percent of American adults were overweight.[2] Things have not improved since these results were recorded. Today, in all, more than two-thirds of adults in the United States are overweight or obese. Why does this matter? Because excess weight impacts health. Conditions directly related to obesity include type 2 diabetes, stroke, heart disease, and certain types of cancer. *These chronic "lifestyle diseases" are some of the leading causes of premature, preventable death.*

The rise in obesity and diabetes is no accident. There's a clear cause: We're eating more processed food than ever before in human history. Obesity rates in the United States in the 1930s were almost nonexistent at less than 1 percent. Now Harvard is predicting that by the year 2030, 50 percent of the U.S. population will be classified as obese.[3]

In 2018, the University of North Carolina at Chapel Hill published a study show-ing that only 1 in 8 Americans are metabolically healthy, which equates to only 12 percent![4] In addition, in 2022 the *Journal of the American College of Cardiology* published a study revealing that 93 percent of American adults are metabolically unhealthy. In other words, only 7 percent of people would be classified as metabolically healthy.[5]

How many people in the United States live a healthy lifestyle? The Mayo Clinic set out to ask this question back in 2016, and they determined that individuals living a healthy lifestyle abided by four key metrics:

1. They didn't smoke.

2. They got sufficient exercise each week (classified as moderate or vigorous activity for at least 150 minutes a week).

3. They ate a healthy diet.

4. Their body fat was less than 20 percent for males and less than 30 percent for females.

It turns out that only 2.7 percent of Americans fit this criteria of a healthy lifestyle.[6]

We are failing at biological life. One in four women are infertile, as are one in three males. As a species, we are literally losing the ability to procreate. Other species that have had this problem ultimately became extinct.

We also aren't living as long as we should. After centuries of steadily increasing lifespans, life expectancy in the United States declined from 78.9 years in 2014 to 78.7 years in 2015, and then down to 78.6 years in 2017.[7] We lag behind other compara-ble high-income nations, where they average a lifespan of 82.3 years. In the United States alone, 50 percent of the population is suffering from a chronic illness.[8] The United States ranks 34th in life expectancy at birth,[9] which means many developing nations are doing better than we are.

According to the CDC, one out of three women and one out of two men are diagnosed with cancer during their lifetime.[10] That's a huge number! What's causing this incredible increase?

It's estimated that 60 percent of Americans are prediabetic or diabetic. Sixty-eight percent of these diabetics end up with heart disease, 16 percent will have a stroke, and 70 percent will have diabetic neuropathy, where their nerves are degenerating.[11] I saw this happen with my dad.[12]

My Pain-to-Purpose Message

My dad followed the Standard American Diet (SAD), and as a result he developed type 2 diabetes. I didn't understand the disease, and I blindly followed the instructions his doctors gave him, which were only based on Western medicine principles.

I remember driving my dad to his doctors' appointments and picking up his insulin and medications for reducing his blood sugar. Every Tuesday, I also took him to the grocery store to purchase the foods recommended by his doctor. At this time, I didn't understand how to read ingredient labels, so I followed the instructions and purchased zero-calorie sodas, whole-grain cereal and cereal bars, instant oatmeal, and many other fake healthy foods for my father. Little did I know that these foods were loaded with artificial ingredients, such as aspartame, sucralose, red dyes, and many others, causing his diabetes to become worse. I then proceeded to fill up his seven-day pillbox for the week.

Year after year, my father's health declined. He gained weight, and the dosage of his medications increased. One day he called me because he was having terrible diabetic neuropathy in his feet, and he was having a hard time walking. My mother and I picked him up and took him to the emergency room. Neuropathy occurs when there's a lack of blood flow to the extremities caused by elevated sugar in the bloodstream. This can be a serious issue because it leads to infection, which could spread to the rest of the body and cause death. To prevent this from happening, doctors often amputate the feet to save the rest of the body. Every 24 hours, 238 amputations take place in the United States in people with diabetes.[13] My father knew an amputation might be in his future.

After being admitted to the emergency room, he experienced high stress thinking about the possibility of losing his feet, and he suffered a massive stroke, which left the entire right side of his body paralyzed. He also lost the ability to speak. The craziest part of this story is that the doctors and nurses didn't know he was having a stroke. I remember walking into the hospital room to check on him, and he wasn't speaking to me. He was just looking at me with such hopeless eyes. I said, "Dad, are you okay? Why aren't you speaking to me?" I knew something was terribly wrong, so I tracked down his doctor and nurses. After several tests, they determined he had suffered a stroke, but it was too late. The damage had been done.

After the stroke, they transferred my dad to hospice care. Week after week, I witnessed his body shrink before my eyes. Nine months into this extremely challenging time, I went to see him one evening. My father was in the worst shape I had ever seen. When I walked into the room, he was convulsing and throwing up on himself.

I immediately flagged down the nurses to help. They cleaned him up, and he looked better. Before I left, I walked up to him and looked him square in the eyes. His eyes were hopeless. I told him how much I loved him. I shared that he would always be my father, and I would always be his son. I kissed him on the forehead and whispered the words, "Hasta la vista, baby." One of our favorite movies was *The Terminator,* and he always quoted that line to me when he said good-bye.

I drove home that night, sobbing the entire time. I remember arriving home and uttering the same prayer I had been saying for weeks, which was to please end my father's suffering. It had been enough, and all I wanted was for him to be at peace. There was something different this time—I felt an energy, a feeling that someone, something, was listening to me. I went to bed, and 12 hours later I received the phone call that my father had passed.

Losing my father raised several questions for me. I wanted to know why he'd had to endure so much pain when we had followed the advice from his doctors. Yet it's not only my father—far too many people are dealing with sickness. Are we designed for sickness? Why is there such an epidemic of disease?

I took a deep dive into the research, and to my surprise, I discovered that my father's doctors were only treating his symptoms. His doctors failed to see that there was a cause and an effect, not just a result. I soon realized that the same information I was teaching on stages all over the world—and now in this book—was the same information that could have saved my father's life. I also knew that I was given that mountain so I could show the world this mountain can be moved. This was my pain-to-purpose message.

Understanding the Cause

Something has to change. We need to recognize that the human body has the innate ability to heal itself and provide these tools for healing. Back in 1858, Dr. Rudolph Virchow, founder of the field of cellular pathology, said all diseases are disturbances at the cellular level. He made the case that to treat any disease, we must first understand the cause, and the cause is always found at the level of the cell. Once you work on removing the cause, and in some cases causes, the disease and symptoms go away by default.

Type 2 diabetes medication will show an improvement in blood sugar levels, but diabetes is getting worse. Conventional medicine treats the symptom (glucose), when the root cause is excessive insulin and cell membrane inflammation. By taking insulin, you make the root cause and the diabetes worse. You can't superficially treat only the symptoms and expect the disease to get better. This is exactly what happened to my dad . . . and what's happening to millions of people. The cell receptor sites have become desensitized to the screams of insulin. Therefore, the beta cells need to work harder and "shout" to get the message across. This is like when you first shout at your child to clean their room. They listen at first, but if you keep shouting at them to clean their room for months and years, they eventually become desensitized and start to ignore you. Medication and insulin may regulate the blood sugar levels, but they'll fail to help you recover your sensitivity.

What is the solution? Ancient healing strategies. A low-carbohydrate, keto lifestyle paired with intermittent fasting (IF) have been proven to help sensitize your cell receptor sites so your pancreas doesn't have to work so hard.[14, 15, 16]

The Science and Art of Metabolism

After working with tens of thousands of people from different walks of life, it became clear to me that *no diet will work if your metabolism has interference.* The main reason why so many people fail to get well these days is because they place their focus on the symptom instead of the cause. The book you hold in your hands will help you identify the interference, so you can remove it and allow your body to heal itself.

Many of my clients have tried to speed up their metabolism by using harmful supplements and extreme approaches, only to find themselves in a worse situation. They have discovered my work because what I offer doesn't rely on willpower; it provides an understanding of how the metabolism works, and simple yet effective steps toward metabolic freedom.

Since 2008, I've delivered keynote lectures across the world on the topic of metabolic flexibility—where you flex in and out of fat burning—and I've developed online courses with step-by-step videos and guides. I have a popular YouTube channel with over 300,000 subscribers and over 20 million video views from people across the globe.

My social media following has grown to over one million combined followers who are eager to learn this information. I'm in the unique position of having interviewed over 900 of the best doctors, scientists, and researchers in the health industry for my *Metabolic Freedom* podcast. I've taken close to 5,000 people through the protocols you're going to learn in this book via my online coaching programs. And I've personally worked one on one with hundreds of clients who had tried almost everything to get well but were still dealing with mystery illnesses. I've been able to teach them how to become health detectives to identify their interferences, remove them, and allow their bodies to heal themselves.

This book is the culmination of my personal and clinical experience, along with my 17-plus years of research. The millions of people who have discovered my work when they were feeling helpless have inspired me to write it. *Metabolic Freedom* is different from anything you've read before because we tie in the science and art of metabolism. I will help you shift from being a sugar burner to a fat burner by gradually decreasing carbohydrates and steadily increasing healthy fats and proteins. This helps alleviate cravings and symptoms, so you will stick with the plan. Once you've shifted to fat-burning mode, I'll pair that with IF, which increases your metabolic efficiency. You will then flex back and forth from fat burning to sugar burning to ensure that your metabolism keeps adapting to change, which is key for results.

In these pages, you'll find proven strategies for restoring your metabolism that I have used to help tens of thousands of people just like you thrive. This book is divided into two key sections. In the first part, we'll explore the primary causes of metabolic dysfunction, delving into the factors that disrupt optimal metabolic health. In the second part, I'll present effective, science-backed solutions to help you restore and revitalize your metabolism. Additionally, you'll find a comprehensive 30-day plan to put these strategies into action, complete with delicious, fat-burning recipes, and a glossary at the end for easy reference.

As you move through the pages of this book, you will learn:

- the main causes of metabolic dysfunction—and the solution for each problem
- how to allow your innate intelligence to work for you to reset your metabolism without feeling restricted or starved
- ancient healing strategies such as ketosis and fasting that teach the body to burn stored fat instead of sugar
- the role of our chemical messengers called hormones and how to keep them balanced
- which foods damage your metabolism and which ones support it
- how your thoughts influence health or disease
- the latest cutting-edge biohacks to double your results in half the amount of time
- how to customize the tools outlined in this book using a 30-Day Metabolic Freedom Reset

You'll realize that there is a path back to perfect health that is unique to you. No matter your stage in life or individual circumstances, this book is designed to help you find your customized path. The best thing about the 30-Day Metabolic Freedom Reset in Chapter 12 is that it's actually easy to follow.

Metabolic Freedom will inspire you to reconnect with your innate intelligence so this inner physician can go to work for you and allow your body to heal itself. Whether you're managing high cholesterol, autoimmune disorders, diabetes, or other metabolic conditions, this book provides the precise steps you need to reclaim your health and restore balance to your life.

I'll be your sherpa, holding your hand gently as you take back control of your health. I'm excited to share in the pages ahead the only solution you'll ever need to reset your metabolism, balance your hormones, and burn fat. The 30-Day Metabolic Freedom Reset seamlessly integrates with any dietary approach you choose, whether you're a meat-eater, vegan, or vegetarian. I hope this book changes your life by helping you identify what has been interfering with your metabolism—so you feel better today, and prevent disease tomorrow.

Let's dive in and uncover how to break free from the cycle of yo-yo dieting, so you can burn fat effectively and feel incredible every day. Get ready for a paradigm shift in health that will serve you in so many incredible ways. I'm writing this with a big smile on my face, because I'm grateful to hold your hand and walk you through the process to achieve metabolic freedom. Hold on to your metabolic hats!

PART I

THE PROBLEMS

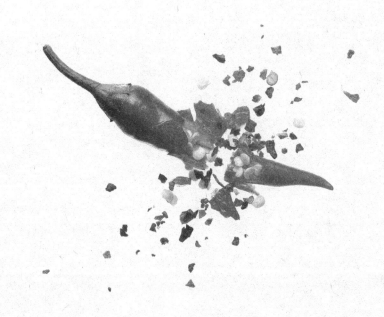

CHAPTER 1

WE NEED A NEW PARADIGM FOR FAT LOSS

At the beginning of my weight-loss journey in 2008, I thought it was as simple as burning more calories than I consumed to achieve my desired fat-loss outcome. My focus was on losing weight to get healthy. I began exercising more and eating less, and the weight started to come off. But then something happened. A few weeks in, I found myself hungrier and having to rely on more willpower and sheer discipline to get through each day. Eventually the fat loss slowed down and then I plateaued. My first thought was to cut my calories even more and burn more calories through exercise. It worked! At least for a couple of weeks . . . until the same problem kept occurring.

I eventually discovered that *being overweight was not my problem—it was my symptom.* By focusing on weight loss and caloric restriction, I was treating the symptom but never getting to the *cause.* This was one of my biggest aha moments, because it led me to discover that nobody has ever had a weight problem. Even when I was obese, I never had a weight problem. It was a weight symptom! When I shifted my focus to hormones and cell inflammation, the symptoms disappeared by default. Many people are focused on their symptoms but never truly get to the cause, which is at the cell level.

In this chapter, I'll reveal the main reason you gained weight and have trouble keeping it off. I'll also dismantle the old theory of your genes determining your destiny. We'll explore why our cells are critical to fat burning and how chronic inflammation can interfere with their ability to function, causing uncomfortable physical symptoms. I'll also share what I call the "five fat-loss failures" and the science behind why they don't work.

Your Cells Help You Burn Fat

Your body has a built-in communication system, governed by your cells, to make sure metabolic fat burning happens effortlessly. Think of this intelligence as an air traffic controller at the airport. Just as an air traffic controller is responsible for making sure hundreds of flights take off and land safely each day, each cell inside your body functions in a similar way, communicating with your hormones so you can burn fat and produce energy.

How many air traffic controllers do you have inside of your body? According to an estimate published in 2013 in the *Annals of Human Biology* by an international team of researchers, and appropriately entitled "An estimation of the number of cells in the human body," you have about 37.2 trillion cells. If lined up, your cells would wrap around the Earth 2 million times. That's a lot of flights![1]

Our internal and external environments affect every one of our cells. The DNA in them gets injured throughout the day, and we must repair our genome (the complete set of genes within a cell) several times a day. With our 20,000 genes, we can build 4 million different variants of ourselves!

Why am I starting a chapter about fat loss by discussing genetics? Because when we're diagnosed with obesity—or even serious conditions such as cancer or heart disease—we're often told that this condition was in our genes. It's not our fault; it was just bad luck. This message is outdated, as you'll see throughout this book. With the lifestyle changes you're about to embark on, you have the power to positively influence your genetic expression, transforming your health at the deepest level.

What if you want to build yourself a new body? Guess what? You can!

We've seen this many times before. When you run into an old friend who suddenly looks completely different—well, they built themselves a different body. You can actually build yourself a new body of vibrant cells within a matter of days, once you give your metabolism the building blocks it needs to thrive. You can also replicate sick cells when you give your metabolism inflammatory, processed foods that are abundant in our food supply. The choice is yours.

The length of a cell's life varies depending on the type. The following table shows the lifespan of various cells.

THE LIFESPAN OF CELLS

Cell Type	Longevity
White blood cells	Approximately 13 days
Skin cells	About 30 days
Red blood cells	Around 120 days
Liver cells	Renewed every 150 to 500 days
	Can regrow even after up to 90 percent removal
Hair cells	6 years (women), 3 years (men)
Stomach/Intestine cells	Up to 5 days
Bones	Osteocytes: Up to 25 years
	Complete regeneration cycle: 10 years
Heart cells	New cells generated throughout lifespan
	Half of birth cells still present at 50 years old
	Replacement slows with age: 1 percent at 25, 0.5 percent at 75
Brain cells	Neurons in cerebral cortex may last a lifetime
	Regeneration of damaged cells possible (neurogenesis)

How Inflammation Interferes with Our Cells

When you pause to think of how magnificent your human body is, you'll find yourself in awe. As you read this sentence, I want you to place your right hand over your right ear and keep it there as I share this with you.

Got it? Okay.

You are a masterpiece because you are a piece of the master. *Your body is not broken.* Your body's a vessel for your beautiful soul. You were designed to thrive while experiencing peak vitality, energy, and vibrance.

Okay, you can remove your hand now. You're probably wondering why I had you place your hand over your ear. I didn't want this message to go in one ear and out the other!

Inside your body is a beautiful orchestra of hormones circulating in your blood. These chemical messengers attach to your cell receptor sites, unlock the cell door, and communicate with the cells themselves. When this happens the way you were designed, you burn fat and feel good—and obesity becomes obsolete. Here's the question: If you were created this way, why are 93 percent of American adults metabolically unhealthy?[2]

Your cells have receptor sites called *integral membrane proteins*. These receptor sites are integrated within each cell, and they act like a cell phone tower. A cell phone tower receives a signal from its environment and performs a job. Your receptor sites receive signals from your hormones, nutrients (both food and supplements), oxygen, and even thoughts. When this communication system is not working properly, symptoms will develop. There's only one main reason why this communication system becomes dysfunctional: because of inflammation. You've likely heard the term *inflammation* before, but it's important to note that there are two types and understand the difference between them.

Acute Inflammation vs. Chronic Inflammation

Acute inflammation is not necessarily bad. As you'll learn in the upcoming pages, there's a benefit to causing short-term stress so your body can become stronger. This is a principle called *hormesis,* which we'll discuss in detail later. Think of acute inflammation as soreness from a workout; your body adapts to the stress, repairs any damage, and recovers, and you become healthier and stronger. Chronic inflammation, on the other hand, is the boogeyman we want to avoid.

Each cell has a lipid (fatty) bilayer wrapped around it called the cell membrane, which is composed of a double layer of phospholipid molecules. The cell membrane functions as the outer "skin" of the cell and controls the passage of materials into and out of it. Proteins in the cell membrane provide various services, including structural support and the formation of channels for the passage of materials. Think of the cell membranes as the bodyguards of your cells.

Scientists once believed that the DNA nucleus served as the intelligence within your cells. But their premise was proven to be flawed when Dr. Bruce Lipton, a world-renowned cell biologist, arrived on the scene. He challenged the notion that your DNA runs the show, conducting experiments where he'd remove the DNA nucleus from cells and observe what would happen next. To his surprise, the cell continued to function without any issues for months. This proved that something else was in charge, so he set out to discover what that was. Dr. Lipton found that when you remove the *cell membrane*, the cell instantly dies, which means that the wisdom inside of our bodies is contained in the cell membrane—it is where life begins and ends.[3, 4]

This brings us back to chronic inflammation. When your cell membrane is chronically inflamed, hormones, amino acids, nutrients, minerals, oxygen, and so on will be blocked from entering the cell. The figure below demonstrates how this looks at the cellular level.

Figure 1. Comparison of unhealthy and healthy cell.

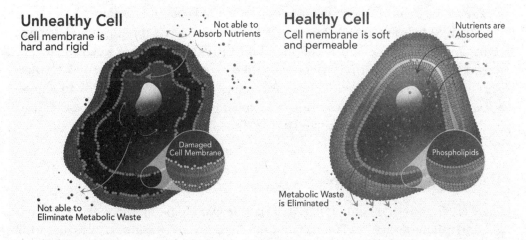

This leads to symptoms. These symptoms start out as general fatigue, brain fog, and weight gain, but if not addressed properly they could lead to diabetes, heart disease, autoimmune disorders, and even cancer.

Symptoms Are Your Body's Check-Engine Light

Your body is smart. When there's interference, it will speak to you. If you were on a long road trip, and suddenly your car's check-engine light turned on, what would you do? Would you ignore it? Would you cover it up with some duct tape and keep on driving? If you chose this option, you'd most likely end up destroying your car, or at the very least crashing it, which would get you into serious trouble. A better option would be to pull over or drive it to a mechanic, pop open the hood, and investigate the interference. Your symptoms are your body's check-engine light—and thank God it has this to show you when you are out of balance.

So when there's interference, the best thing to do is find out where that interference is coming from. Conventional medicine, however, chooses to chase symptoms instead of investigate their source. For example, let's say you went out and gorged yourself one night. You consumed the following: an entire pizza, a full plate of spaghetti and meatballs, four beers, and two scoops of ice cream.

You woke up the next morning with the following symptoms: a headache, gas, bloating, indigestion, and acid reflux. You scheduled an appointment with your conventional doctor. You explained your numerous symptoms, and your doctor prescribed numerous medications, including an antacid and an antidiuretic.

Are those symptoms the problem or are they your feedback mechanisms? What if your doctor instead asked the question, "What did you eat last night?"

Again, symptoms are a beautiful gift from your innate intelligence. The most common symptoms linked to cell membrane inflammation are weight gain and weight-loss resistance. This is why trendy diets have failed you. Most quick-fix diets work against the way you were designed at the cell level, making it difficult to achieve results that stick. In the next section, I'll explain why most diet programs fail: they focus on treating symptoms rather than addressing the root causes.

The Five Fat-Loss Failures

There are five myths about fat loss that have led you to being frustrated with your results. I call these the "five fat-loss failures." These myths encompass ideas like using snacks to boost metabolism, believing carbohydrates are crucial for fat loss, the notion of calories in versus calories out, the reliance on willpower, and the belief in one-size-fits-all approaches.

Before I reveal the specifics, I want you to know that *the failure of your previous attempts to lose weight is not your fault*. Weight loss is a big business for four reasons:

1. Many people want to lose weight.
2. They sign up for expensive weight-loss programs.
3. The programs fail.
4. They repeat the process over and over again.

The problem is that most programs—and even doctors, dietitians, and nutritionists—promote *losing weight to get healthy.* This is not how the body works. We don't lose weight to get healthy; *we get healthy to lose weight.*

The "lose weight to get healthy" approach creates a vicious cycle. A person steps on the scale and says, "I need to lose 50 pounds." They sign up for one of dozens of diet plans. They do the plan and lose some weight. But the plan is painful, and after a while, they give up and return to their old habits. The weight returns. They step on the scale and say, "I need to lose 50 pounds . . . again." So, they sign up for another diet. Around and around it goes like *Groundhog Day* but without the happy ending.

Part of the problem is that the mechanisms of weight control are very complicated and susceptible to wild theories. This lack of understanding leads to the proliferation of "solutions" that don't lead to positive outcomes.

For example, if a cell membrane is inflamed, the fat-burning hormones t3, leptin, testosterone, and human growth hormone won't be able to enter it to communicate the message to "burn fat." It's like joining a Zoom meeting with your co-workers when your mic is muted. Your co-workers can't hear you, so you speak louder until you're screaming; eventually, you get frustrated (and maybe fired). This is what trendy fad diets end up doing: simply frustrate you. If you had been told, "Hey, your mic is muted," then you could have simply unmuted it. This book will teach you how to unmute your cells, so they receive the fat-burning message, and no one has to get fired. Well, maybe Big Pharma and Big Food.

Let's take a close look at each of these five fat-loss failures.

1. Calories In vs. Calories Out

Most traditional diets fail because of weight regain. We can learn a lot about the flaws with this method from the television show *The Biggest Loser.* If you recall, the contestants on this popular TV show were all obese. They were assigned personal trainers who focused on the "calories in vs. calories out" method of weight loss. The participants increased their exercise and decreased their caloric intake. It sounds logical, doesn't it? This concept is based on the idea that as long as you consume fewer calories than you burn, you're bound to lose weight. The problem is that this is much too simplistic and does not take into account real-life conditions.

The participants achieved incredible results during the recording of the show, highlighted and applauded on the final episode. Yet in a 2016 study in the journal *Obesity,* of the 14 contestants researchers followed, 13 of them regained at least some of the weight they had lost during the competition, and over the following six years, 5 were above their pre-competition weight. The contestants featured in the study had regained an average of 90 pounds (70 percent of their lost weight); they also were hungrier with an even slower metabolism than when they started the show! It turns out that the contestants' leptin levels—a hormone that signals to your brain that you're full, so put down the fork—had plummeted after the show and never recovered. This is why there's never been a *Biggest Loser* reunion show![5]

Although this is an extreme example, I see variations of this happening to many people who try popular weight-loss diets. Calories matter, but they aren't that important. When I owned a gym in Miami back in 2013, I hosted seminars on the science of fat loss. I would teach the members of my gym to calculate how many calories they burned each day, and then I'd place them in a calorie deficit. It worked . . . in the beginning. It failed in the long run, which confirmed my hypothesis that what is more important than the *quantity* of calories we consume is the *quality* of those calories. I realized that focusing on calories was a huge distraction from what really matters: hormones and inflammation.

The fact is that in terms of their effects on the human body, not all calories are *processed* equally. They come "packaged" in different foods, and how these foods are digested makes a huge difference in both how the calories are absorbed and how much they satiate your appetite. This means that the calories from sugary foods like cookies are instantly digested, converted into glucose, and absorbed into your bloodstream, causing your blood sugar levels to spike sharply. Your brain receives a huge surge of a feel-good chemical called dopamine. Then when your blood sugar levels drop as your cells absorb the glucose, you may feel jittery and anxious—the "sugar crash." Prolonged consumption of sugar has been linked to a greater risk of depression. It leaves you metabolically handcuffed to your next meal or snack.

In contrast, when you eat salmon, your digestive system has to work to free the calories locked in the proteins and fat. The calories are released and introduced into your bloodstream slowly, over time. This keeps your blood sugar levels stable, and the fat keeps you feeling full and satiated.

Getting the majority of your calories from carbohydrates is unhealthy—but that's exactly what too many Americans do. Concerning overall caloric intake, carbohydrates comprise around 55 percent of the typical American diet, ranging from 200 to 350 grams per day. The vast potential of refined carbohydrates to cause harmful effects is stunning: A greater intake of sugar-laden food is associated with a 44 percent increased prevalence of metabolic syndrome and obesity and a 26 percent increase in the risk of developing diabetes mellitus.[6]

Let's be clear: Calories play a role, but it's much smaller than people think. Calories, which are the measurement of potential energy, are calculated with an automatic buffer zone that's conducted in a very controlled environment in a laboratory and does not factor in the body's complex system. For example, a carbohydrate has 4 calories in the lab, but it can be 3 or 5 calories inside the body. It's almost impossible to count calories from meals once those calories enter our digestive system.

The body isn't a linear system, like the laws of thermodynamics; rather, it is an open system with several variables. It is a demand-driven machine, not a supply-driven machine. Hormones and inflammatory levels determine the demand. *Hormones trump calories every single time.* For example, when the energy sensors insulin and mTOR (mechanistic target of rapamycin) are activated from carbohydrates, our body turns on its anabolic state, which builds muscle and stores fat. When we eat more fat and fewer carbohydrates, our metabolism lowers insulin and mTOR and activates the sympathetic tone (healthy stress response) and autophagy (cell recycling). This signals the breakdown of body fat and muscle, and the body is now in repair mode. This is when fat-burning is activated, controlled by hormones not calories.

Recent studies have investigated the impact of fecal microbiota transplantation (FMT) on weight loss, revealing intriguing findings. One study conducted a randomized controlled trial in which participants with obesity received FMT from lean donors while maintaining their caloric intake. Despite no significant changes in gut hormones such as glucagon-like peptide-1 (GLP-1), which regulates satiety, recipients of the fecal transplant showed notable alterations in their gut microbiota. These changes were associated with a decrease in specific bile acids and increased microbial diversity, leading to modest weight loss and improved metabolic markers even without changes in diet or caloric intake.[7, 8, 9]

The key concept to remember, which we will return to many times in this book, is that we are genetically hardwired for the way our ancestors ate for thousands of years. Until very recently—really, just the past 50 years or so—the human digestive system was accustomed to a diet high in natural fats, fiber, and protein, and low in carbohydrates. This was the nutrient mix it successfully utilized. Sugar was in the form of fructose from fruit, which was bound up in fiber and took a long time to extract. Sure, our lifestyle is dramatically different from that of our ancestors. We no longer spend all day hunting for our next meal. However, our metabolism doesn't recognize the difference between intentionally skipping a meal for intermittent fasting and experiencing a famine.

It's time to stop distracting ourselves by focusing on calories in vs calories out. If you asked Warren Buffet, "How do you get rich?" and he answered, "Easy—spend less than you earn," you wouldn't feel good about his answer, would you? This is the same with doctors, dietitians, and fitness pros telling people to simply eat less and move more. Focusing on calories is the opposite of metabolic freedom. It distracts you from what really matters: hormones and cell metabolism.

2. Eat Lots of Small Meals All Day

As we'll discuss later in the book, how *often* we eat is just as important as *what* we eat. For most of human history, food was available only intermittently during the day. When you were working in the fields, you couldn't stop for a "snack." You filled your belly at mealtime, worked for many hours, and then took another meal. It was common for healthy people to go without food for 12 hours or more at a time— typically from dinner until breakfast the next day. Food had to be rationed, especially during the winter when your food supply was limited to only protein and fat. There was nothing unusual about this; it was simply the normal routine. There were no refrigerators stocked with fresh food, no Taco Bell open at midnight, and no 24-hour restaurants. When the sun set, your outside labor ceased, and you rested until dawn.

Even though we are still genetically hardwired like our ancestors, today we see many health "gurus," nutritionists, and dietitians advising people to practice portion control, cut calories, and eat every two or three hours. They say this strategy of "grazing" will help you lose weight and keep your metabolism "revved up."

Are they right? Somewhat yes, but mostly no.

In the short term, this may appear to work, but in the long term, it has a 99 percent failure rate. Here's just one problem with grazing: If you want to age faster than anyone else in your neighborhood, then eat every two or three hours. When you constantly consume calories, your body starts to duplicate its cells. This is great for a growing child but bad for a grown adult. Accelerated cell division is the essence of aging. You'll learn later in the book about how your metabolism does not work in terms of speeds—it's either efficient or inefficient.

Furthermore, many diseases start in the gut. If you're grazing and constantly have food in your stomach, you're not allowing your digestive system to rest. Some of the major contributors to digestive disorders like heartburn, indigestion, and food intolerance are underlying metabolic problems, including lack of enzymes, intolerance to foods, chemical toxicity, and chronic constipation. Many of these symptoms are caused by eating too frequently. Eating meals too often does not allow the body enough time to recuperate between meals and reload its enzyme pool. This can cause a lack of enzymes and hydrochloric acid in the stomach, leading to the development of digestive disorders with conditions such as acid reflux (heartburn), esophageal disorders and cancer, and food intolerance.[10]

In a fascinating study conducted at the University of Virginia, researchers took a group of college students and fed them 800 calories of pizza from a local restaurant popular with the students, and tracked how much stress this meal caused within the digestive tract. What they discovered was astounding. Fourteen hours after eating, this meal was *not* fully digested—and keep in mind that younger people typically have a faster digestive system!

When you eat meals frequently throughout the day, especially processed high-carbohydrate meals (typical SAD fare), it destroys the gut integrity at the tight junction—the level of the lining of the gut that affects how cells are held together.

In a healthy gut, cells are closely linked by structures called *tight junctions*. These junctions act like gatekeepers, letting nutrients pass through to the bloodstream while keeping harmful substances out. If the tight junctions are weakened or damaged, the gut lining becomes "leaky," allowing unwanted particles—like bacteria, toxins, and undigested food—to pass into the bloodstream. This is often referred to as *leaky gut syndrome*.

This breakdown in gut integrity can lead to inflammation and trigger immune responses, potentially contributing to various health issues, including food sensitivities, autoimmune conditions, and metabolic problems.

What happens next? The liver becomes inflamed and then changes the hormonal cascade. The liver has a major role in the endocrine system. When you stress it, you can develop fatty liver syndrome very quickly. Fatty liver is when too much fat builds up in the liver, making it harder for the liver to do its job of filtering toxins and producing energy. This buildup can lead to inflammation and, over time, cause liver damage if not addressed. Inflammatory genes cascade through the entire system, the blood-brain barrier breaks down, the kidneys stop filtering well, and you become a sponge for toxins and inflammation. Chronic digestive stress leads to digestive and autoimmune disorders.

As you'll learn later in the book when we cover ketosis, when you use fat as the primary fuel source, it burns very cleanly, as opposed to burning sugar, which is a "dirty" fuel source. Glucose burns quickly and easily, but it also burns dirty via excessive production of free radicals. Think of burning fat as a natural gas stove and burning sugar (glucose) as burning firewood. The gas stove burns clean with no smoke; the firewood creates massive amounts of toxic smoke.

Free radicals are highly unstable molecules with one or more unpaired electrons in their outer shells. They are formed from molecules via the breakage of a chemical bond, such that each fragment keeps one electron. They are produced either from normal cell metabolism or from external sources, including radiation, pollution, medication, and cigarette smoke. Since they can be either harmful or helpful to the body, they play a dual role as both toxic and beneficial compounds. But when an excess of free radicals cannot be removed, their accumulation in the body generates a phenomenon called *oxidative stress*. Excessive free radicals are the driving force behind inflammation, cancer, and accelerated aging.

Grazing promotes the production of free radicals, which in excess are harmful and promote aging. I receive a lot of backlash from the fitness community when I say that eating every two to three hours will age you faster, but it's the truth!

The secret to perfect health is in mimicking the eating behaviors of our hunter-gatherer ancestors. Science is showing that intermittent fasting enhances the body's resistance to oxidative stress and helps fight inflammation, another key driver of many common diseases.[11] I will teach you more about the science and art of IF in Chapter 8.

In short, give your stomach a rest! Let it be empty for several hours a day, which aligns with the way your digestive system was created. This is the first step in going from bad health to good health and from despair to hope.

3. The Metabolism Needs Carbohydrates to Burn Fat and Function

This is false. You don't need to consume glucose from carbohydrates in your diet. Your body *makes* glucose, and you get all the sugar you require by burning your excess body fat and from the protein you eat. The medical term is *gluconeogenesis*, and it is the metabolic process by which organisms produce sugars (glucose) for catabolic reactions from non-carbohydrate precursors. Essentially, your own body fat combined with amino acids from the proteins you eat keep blood sugars at homeostasis. The body uses insulin to tightly control blood sugar levels, so that at any given time, less than one little teaspoon of sugar is in your entire bloodstream. As the *British Journal of Nutrition* reveals, even with prolonged fasting, and drinking only water, blood glucose levels in the average healthy adult will remain stable.[12]

Proteins are a source of gluconeogenic substances, which under fasting or a low-carbohydrate intake can be used to produce glucose. High-protein (HP) diets are generally low in carbohydrates and are assumed to promote gluconeogenesis after a meal. Again, your body has all the glucose it needs to burn fat, so your metabolism doesn't require additional carbohydrates.

4. One-Size-Fits-All Approaches

Most diets work—just not long term. I share this onstage often when delivering keynote lectures, which always shocks my audience.

When people first begin a weight-loss diet, they're usually gung-ho, and it may be easy for them to make low-calorie meals or keep their refrigerator stocked with healthy food. But as the weeks and months drag on, their previous behavior returns. They see their diet as punitive and start to "cheat." Or they think, "Great! I've lost weight. I should reward myself for enduring this torture." To lose weight and enjoy good health, people need to make a total lifestyle change, not just follow a diet.

Diets have an end date. Your health is a lifelong journey.

Restrictive dieting often means going against your body's stubborn instinct to maintain your weight. This trait evolved in humans from long ago when food was scarcer and took more effort to acquire. By cutting out foods your body craves—particularly fats—you're fighting nature and setting yourself up for failure. If you're told not to eat things that you like, for the first few days you can resist eating them. But then your primal brain will start taking over, and you'll want what you can't have.

We also all have different hormonal needs at different times of our lives, and our diet needs to sync up with this. As you'll learn in the coming chapters, there's an art to fat loss, which all weight-loss diets fail to teach. I'm going to educate you on how different hormones influence mood, satiety, and weight loss—and how to customize your nutrition to optimize these hormones. The magic happens when you find a lifestyle customized to your hormones. This brings me to the last fat-loss failure.

5. Relying on Willpower to Lose Weight

The fact that you're reading this book suggests that you've decided to do something about your health. Perhaps you want to finally put an end to yo-yo weight loss. You may be worried about your symptoms becoming worse and leading to heart disease, cancer, or one of the other severe medical conditions linked to poor metabolic health. Maybe you want to set an example for your children, so they don't have to experience the same suffering.

Unlike other methods, the *Metabolic Freedom* road map does not require willpower. Most people fail to achieve sustainable fat loss because they've had these bad habits for decades, and they have reasons they won't give them up. It can also be hard when you choose to make changes and people inside your own home are not on board, not to mention when you go out to an event or a trip, which provides unique challenges to maintaining new habits.

The problem with most fat-loss plans is that they make you change too many things at once. This requires you to rely on willpower. Not only is this not sustainable, but also all these changes disrupt your household, because your partner sees the extreme, rapid changes you're making, and they may not like it. What I have found while working with thousands of people across the world, is that when you have a dedicated, easy-to-follow plan, you can make a clean break from the past, without feeling deprived or requiring any willpower.

The 30-Day Metabolic Freedom Reset, which you'll find in Chapter 12, is designed to help your household support you because there are no extreme changes being made. Most couples will support each other for 30 days, especially when it's not an extreme plan. Maybe your partner will even join you.

It's time to let go of self-limiting beliefs and the five fat-loss failures that have brainwashed us and step into a new possibility. You have the power. Within every cell of your body is an ancient intelligence that no doctor, pill, surgery, or supplement can match. This journey will require you to believe you can do this.

Forget about the past, and any setbacks you've had. It's not about the setbacks; it's about the getbacks! I believe setbacks are setups for something great. It's not your fault that you've been fed a handful of lies about your body. Let go of the past—it doesn't serve you. Once you make this decision, you open a door of possibility beyond your wildest dreams.

Now it's time to dive deeper into the heart of the matter: understanding how your metabolism actually works. This isn't just science; it's the blueprint that will empower you to take real, lasting control over your health. I've found that the more clearly we understand something, the easier it becomes to apply that knowledge in a way that's meaningful and sustainable. And I'm confident this will be the same for you. When we truly understand our metabolism, we open the door to choices that restore balance, energy, and vitality.

CHAPTER 2

MISUNDERSTANDING HOW YOUR METABOLISM WORKS

One of the most amazing things about your body is the way your metabolism works. It doesn't necessarily operate by speed—it operates by efficiency or inefficiency. An efficient metabolism has the ability to extract energy from whatever substance is available for the job at hand. For example, your metabolism can create energy from the fat stores in your body, the calories on your plate of food, the glycogen stores inside your liver and muscle cells, the glucose in your bloodstream, and the ketone bodies your liver makes in the absence of glucose. When you are metabolically free, your metabolism can use any of these methods without you even noticing.

If we examine the lifestyle of our hunter-gatherer ancestors, we find evidence that being metabolically flexible kept people from going extinct. Our ancestors didn't know where their next meal was coming from (or when they'd get it), so their metabolism became fine-tuned to use whatever was available for energy. Our metabolism is still hardwired this way.

Unfortunately, only 7 percent of people in the United States have a healthy, flexible metabolism in the way I just described. As I referenced in the Introduction, 93 percent of people in the United States are metabolically handcuffed. Their metabolism is only efficient at using one of the available energy methods: glucose (sugar). There's nothing wrong with using glucose as an energy source, unless it's your only energy source.

In this chapter you'll learn some of the incredible healing benefits of a healthy metabolism, such as regenerating the neurons in your brain or repairing your gut microbiome. I'll also share some of the conditions metabolic flexibility works best for, such as breaking weight-loss resistance, helping your body detoxify, and even preventing cancer. Once you understand the science of how your metabolism works, it becomes so much easier to become metabolically healthy.

The Five Healing Benefits of a Flexible Metabolism

When you're metabolically flexible, your body has multiple ways to generate energy and burn fat. In contrast, someone who is metabolically restricted has far fewer options available. Earlier in the book, I shared some scary statistics on cancer, heart disease, diabetes, and many more chronic health conditions. There are five major healing benefits of a flexible metabolism that can help you avoid becoming one of those statistics:

1. creating adaptation through hormetic stress
2. alternating between the repair pathway (autophagy) and growth pathway (mTOR)
3. supporting your mitochondria
4. regenerating neurons in your brain
5. repairing the gut microbiome by creating biodiversity

Let's go through them, one by one.

1. Creating Adaptation through Hormetic Stress

One of the most important principles I have learned about health is called *hormesis*. It will change the way you think about health. Hormesis is defined as a phenomenon in which a harmful substance gives stimulating and beneficial effects to living organisms when the quantity of the harmful substance is small.[1]

Figure 2. How hormesis works.

THE HORMETIC ZONE

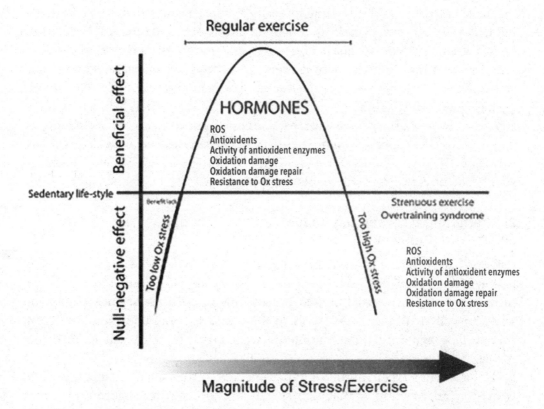

Exercise is the easiest example of how hormesis works. Let's say you've been sedentary for 10 years, and you hear about the benefits of CrossFit. CrossFit is a 60-minute, high-intensity workout often involving Olympic lifts, burst training, and other functional modalities. If you decide that your first workout back into the world of fitness will be a CrossFit one, your body will have a hard time adapting to this stress, you'll be sore for days, and you may even hurt yourself. You'd have done too much and fallen out of your hormetic zone. However, if you instead did a 45-minute walk and some push-ups, squats, and planks, your body most likely could adapt to this light stress, you'd stay within your hormetic zone, and you'd grow stronger and healthier. You'd have found your sweet spot! Over time the goal is to create a higher hormetic ceiling, so you can apply more stressors and stay within the zone of benefits.

Fasting and ketosis are another example. Yes, fasting stresses your body, but it's only a bad stress when you don't properly adapt to the stress. Imagine I'm holding two cups of water. One cup is filled to the brim, while the other is only a quarter full. If I shake both cups with the same intensity—representing stress—the cup that's full will spill water everywhere, symbolizing the onset of symptoms. On the other hand, the cup that's only a quarter full won't spill, even if shaken more vigorously. This illustrates the difference between someone whose stress capacity is maxed out versus someone with less accumulated stress. The person whose cup is filled to the top has a low hormetic ceiling, meaning they can tolerate less stress before symptoms appear. Conversely, the person with the quarter-full cup has a higher hormetic ceiling, allowing them to handle more stress without negative effects. This also explains why some people feel better during fasting, while others do not. When you stay in your hormetic zone, you achieve incredible results.

2. Alternating between the Repair Pathway (Autophagy) and Growth Pathway (mTOR)

Cells are like groceries: When they expire, they need to be thrown out—up to 330 billion of them every day![2] Yet sometimes we have cells within our body that begin to dysfunction, and they stick around. Because they refuse to die, scientists call them senescent cells. I call them *zombie cells*. As they build up in our body, studies suggest they promote aging and the conditions associated with it, such as osteoporosis and Alzheimer's disease.[3, 4, 5]

Zombie cells start out normal but then encounter stress, such as damage to their DNA or a viral infection. At that point, a cell can choose to die or become a zombie, basically entering a state of suspended animation. The problem is that zombie cells release chemicals that can harm nearby normal cells. That's where the trouble starts.

Researchers have also shown that transplanting zombie cells into young mice basically made them act older: their maximum walking speed slowed down, and their muscle strength and endurance decreased.[6] Tests revealed that the implanted cells converted other cells to zombie status.

One of the best ways to kill off these zombie cells is a process called *autophagy*.

Autophagy literally means "eat thyself," and it cleans up damaged cells. Think of the groceries in your refrigerator. What would happen if you allowed them to expire, and instead of throwing the expired food in the trash, you pushed them toward the back of the fridge? You'd create a toxic environment! Mold and bacteria would grow, and many other disgusting processes would occur. Well, your body is just like your refrigerator, in that its cells, fats, and proteins all have expiration dates. If you aren't intentionally "taking out the trash" within your body, this toxic buildup can lead to diseases like cancer and Alzheimer's. Fasting helps your body get rid of these expired products, because it triggers the process of autophagy, which breaks down and recycles dysfunctional proteins and cellular debris.

The opposite of autophagy is a pathway called mTOR, which is short for mechanistic target of rapamycin. This pathway signals growth—it is anabolic. (Think of bodybuilders; they get a ton of mTOR.) This pathway can be healing in spurts, but it can lead to problems if you're in a constant growth state, such as the duplication of these zombie cells. There's an art to balancing autophagy and mTOR, and this is the focus of your 30-Day Metabolic Freedom Reset. As you'll see in the pages ahead, when used as part of the *Metabolic Freedom* lifestyle, intermittent, deliberate fasting can be an easy way to clean out your reserves of glucose, burn ketones, lose weight, and feel great.

3. Supporting Your Mitochondria

The mitochondria are so important that the cells most critical for survival (in terms of energy production needs)—the cells required to stay alive and alert—have the most of them. According to some estimates, each heart muscle cell contains between 5,000 and 8,000 mitochondria, and each neuron can have up to two million!

Mitochondria are also central in retinal cell function and survival. Retinal neurons have high energy requirements, since large amounts of adenosine triphosphate (ATP) are needed to generate membrane potentials and power membrane pumps. Think of ATP as the energy currency created by the mitochondria. In photoreceptors, the number can be quite high as well, with estimates suggesting thousands of mitochondria per cell. The exact number can vary, but it's not uncommon for a single retinal cell, especially a cone photoreceptor, to contain several hundred to a few thousand mitochondria.[7] Compare this to other cells, which have hundreds to a few thousand per cell.

This all makes sense from a survival standpoint. The brain and eyes are required to think and see efficiently so you can capture food for survival or run away from a predator to stay alive. The name of the game is survival!

TEN FASCINATING FACTS ABOUT MITOCHONDRIA

1. You get all of your mitochondria exclusively from your mother.

2. The cells that are most metabolically active, and needed for survival, have the highest concentration of mitochondria.

3. The mitochondria fuse together and communicate (adrenals talk to the brain, etc.). This means your mitochondria from various cells communicate with each other.

4. They produce 95 percent of your body's energy.

5. By age 70, we lose an estimated 56 to 70 percent of mitochondria.

6. Every cell has mitochondria except red blood cells. Red blood cells transport oxygen throughout the body. If they had mitochondria, they would consume some of that oxygen, reducing delivery efficiency to tissues.

7. In one aspect, mitochondria are technically alien organisms inside our bodies. They possess their own DNA (called mtDNA), giving them an independent genome. They operate much like bacteria, but the kind of bacteria working in harmony with our cells in a mutually beneficial symbiotic relationship.

8. The inner mitochondrial membrane contains an unusually high percentage (greater than 70 percent) of proteins, which are involved in oxidative phosphorylation as well as in the transport of metabolites (e.g., pyruvate and fatty acids) between the cytosol (the fluid inside the cell) and mitochondria. Oxidative phosphorylation is the process in which cells produce energy in the mitochondria by using oxygen to convert food into ATP, the energy currency of the cell.

9. The two primary fuels for the mitochondria are minerals and amino acids. The body makes amino acids but not minerals. All these minerals need to come from food sources.

10. There are only two antioxidants the mitochondria can use: glutathione and melatonin.

The mitochondria are much more than "mindless energy factories." Yes, it is important for them to receive energy in the form of glucose, fatty acids, and amino acids, and to produce ATP, but the mitochondria are also highly intelligent. For example, they act like a surveillance system, looking to identify threats.

Cellular threats come in the form of three key areas:

1. mental/emotional
2. physical
3. chemical

The number one priority for the human body is survival. When your "stress bucket" is full, the mitochondria strategically produce less energy, all for the sake of survival. This is called the cell danger response (CDR). The CDR is the evolutionarily conserved metabolic response that protects cells and hosts from harm. It's triggered by encounters with chemical, physical, or biological threats that exceed the cellular capacity for homeostasis. The resulting metabolic mismatch between available resources and functional capacity produces a cascade of changes in cellular function.

When the CDR persists abnormally, whole body metabolism and the gut microbiome are disturbed, the collective performance of multiple organ systems is impaired, behavior is changed, and chronic disease results. Metabolic memory of past stress encounters is stored in the form of altered mitochondrial and cellular macromolecule content, resulting in an increase in functional reserve capacity through a process known as mitocellular hormesis.[8] In simple terms, metabolic memory means that your cells and mitochondria remember past stress, which changes how they function. This memory helps them build up a stronger ability to handle future stress, a process called *mitocellular hormesis*.

As you can see, having a flexible metabolism that supports your mitochondria is a major health benefit.

4. Regenerating Neurons in Your Brain

Your brain also thrives when you are metabolically flexible. Your neurons—the messengers of your brain that communicate every second—get damaged from excess sugar. When you lower glucose levels in the body with ketosis and fasting, you begin to repair these neurons, allowing information to move efficiently from one neuron to the next. This means less brain fog and more mental clarity and energy.

Your brain consists of between 86 and 100 billion neurons, which are the specialized cells that "do the thinking" and create tiny electrical charges. In addition, there are about an equal number of glial cells that maintain homeostasis, form the fatty myelin insulation around the wire-like dendrites that connect the neurons (yet another example of the vital importance of fat), and provide support and protection for neurons.

The fuels that power your brain are glucose, ketones, and oxygen, via the bloodstream. Like other cells in the body, the respiration process in the brain cells creates waste or by-products, including carbon dioxide, water, ammonia, and various types of proteins. In the brain, two proteins in particular are produced: amyloid beta and tau. Amyloid beta is what forms the plaques found in the brains of Alzheimer's patients. Tau, which resembles sets of parallel railroad tracks, can be damaged or "tangled" and cause mitochondrial dysfunction. Tangles of tau are the hallmark of many neurodegenerative diseases. In certain diseases, neurons and/or other brain and nerve cells can have a problem with transporting glucose into the cell and essentially starve and die. Ketones can be taken up by neurons that cannot use glucose.

5. Repairing the Gut Microbiome by Creating Biodiversity

Research has shown that fasting heals the gut. Many of the positive changes that occur in your gut microbiome come to a screeching halt once you eat. We usually think of food as giving us energy, but digesting the food we eat actually *requires* energy. When we eat food, it takes massive amounts of energy to process that food. It is estimated that after a heavy meal, 65 percent of the body's energy must be directed to the digestive organs. During fasting, we rest our system from the constant onslaught of food. We redirect our energy toward healing and recuperation. Our body can detox, repair cells, and eliminate foreign toxins and natural metabolic wastes.

Chewing food and allowing the body to take macronutrients and assimilate them into micronutrients for distribution is a big task. One of my favorite benefits of fasting is a process I call *energy diversion*. When you're in a fasted state, your metabolism diverts resources that would have been used for digestion and directs them toward areas of your body that need healing.

The gut bacteria *Akkermansia* has also been shown to have anti-obesity protective effects, and many companies are now adding it to their probiotics. While the research on whether or not these probiotics can raise this useful bacteria is questionable, studies have shown that fasting increases an abundance of *Akkermansia*.[9] Researchers found that intermittent fasting positively influences the gut microbiome by increasing the diversity of beneficial bacteria while reducing harmful ones. These changes in the gut microbiota were also associated with improvements in blood lipid profiles, suggesting that IF can contribute to better overall metabolic health. The findings highlight the potential of IF as a noninvasive strategy to modulate gut health and improve cardiovascular risk factors.[10]

Five Conditions Metabolic Freedom Supports

Now that you understand how these principles heal your body, let's look at which specific conditions they work best for. There are five distinct times when flexing in and out of fat burning versus sugar burning will be the answer to your health symptoms. Metabolic freedom can support you in:

1. breaking weight-loss resistance
2. preventing cancer
3. slowing the aging process
4. reversing autoimmune conditions
5. detoxifying your body

Let's explore each one of these now.

1. Breaking Weight-Loss Resistance

Survival is the number one priority for your innate intelligence. When you eat, which raises your blood glucose levels, your cells will burn energy from the food you ingested. Anything in excess goes into your glycogen stores, and then is stored in body fat. We'll call this the fed state. When you fast, you turn on a switch that allows your body to tap into your glycogen stores and body fat. We'll call this the fasted state.

When you're looking for lasting weight loss, it's important to train your body to be really efficient at both of these processes. If you spend too much time in the fed state, you remain sugar burning, which signals to your metabolism "keep storing fat." When you spend too much time in the fasted state, your metabolism can see this as a threat to survival, so it slows metabolic rate and weakens your immune system.

The magic is in the adaptation. World-class personal trainers and fitness coaches understand how this works—they are constantly creating different workout routines for their clients because they know that if they keep the muscles adapting to changes, the body achieves better results. This same principle can be applied to your metabolism. When you master the art of switching back and forth between the fed and fasted state, this adaptation creates lasting results. This is how I have helped thousands of people break weight-loss resistance.

2. Preventing Cancer

Whether we "get cancer" is in part (but not always) a result of factors that are due to cellular changes that get "turned on" or "turned off" by behavior that is within our own control, namely: not smoking; eating a healthy, whole-foods diet; and practicing stress-coping mechanisms, including getting enough sleep. We used to think that cancer was the result of an unlucky genetic lottery, and that once you got it there was nothing you could do about it. But there is an interplay between the pro-cancer and anti-cancer events in the body.

The immune system orchestrates what happens when a cell dies and needs to be carted away or grows too rapidly and needs to be neutralized. Anything that strengthens our immune systems is an anti-cancer factor, since our immune system is our first line of defense against runaway cells. On the other hand, anything that inflames our bodies, hampers our immunity, and contributes to the overzealous growth of cells can contribute to the growth of cancer. This includes a diet high in processed carbohydrates and seed oils and simply too much food, in the form of eating larger portions and more food more frequently throughout the day.

Cancer grew in the United States by 84 percent from 1969 until 2014 and only took a minor dip in the intervening years due to smoking cessation trends.[11] Once lung cancer retreated, the statistics on cancer began to look better, but other than smoking, which accounts for 35 percent of attributable risk for cancer, the second largest risk factor is obesity. People who have type 2 diabetes and are overweight have an 18 percent higher risk of cancer than those without type 2 diabetes or obesity.[12] The connection is simple: insulin is a growth hormone. It's one of several nutrient sensors that, when we eat, urge the cells to grow.

If you're eating several snacks and meals throughout the day, then you're constantly signaling the body to grow and grow and grow. When you eat macronutrients, especially carbs, that signals insulin. When you eat protein, that activates another nutrient sensor called mTOR, which is essential for protein synthesis. A third nutrient sense called AMPK responds to all three macronutrients—carbs, protein, and fat—and works long term. In each case, when you keep feeding your body 10 times a day, you're telling the body to grow!

Researchers at the University of California, San Diego, reported that intermittent fasting reduced the risk of breast cancer in obese mice.[13] They found that restricting eating to an eight-hour window, when activity was highest, decreased the risk of development, growth, and metastasis of breast cancer in mice. The findings, published in *Nature Communications*, demonstrated how time-restricted feeding, which is a form of IF, aligned with the circadian rhythms of the subjects and improved metabolic health and tumor circadian rhythms in mice with obesity-driven postmenopausal breast cancer.

"Previous research has shown that obesity increases the risk of a variety of cancers by negatively affecting how the body reacts to insulin levels and changing circadian rhythms," said senior author Nicholas Webster, Ph.D., professor at UC San Diego School of Medicine. "We were able to increase insulin sensitivity, reduce hyperinsulinemia, restore circadian rhythms, and reduce tumor growth by simply modifying when and for how long mice had access to food."

As we've seen before, elevated levels of insulin are damaging to the body. Research data indicated that elevated insulin levels in obese mice drove accelerated tumor growth. Artificially elevated insulin levels accelerated tumor growth, whereas reducing insulin levels could mimic the effect of the time-restricted feeding.[14]

Metabolic flexibility keeps insulin in check, slows cell growth, and helps prevent cancer.

3. Slowing the Aging Process

Although Father Time remains undefeated, the speed at which you age can be slowed down. The key to aging gracefully is to ensure that you remove what is interfering with your metabolism and give your cells all the necessary resources to function optimally. Supporting your cells, specifically your mitochondria, is the name of the game.

Your mitochondria love ketones. Ketones signal to your mitochondria to engage in mitochondrial biogenesis, the creation of new, healthy mitochondria. (I will teach you during the 30-Day Metabolic Freedom Reset which foods to eat to help your body produce ketones.)

Another way to improve mitochondrial function is to stress it (remember hormesis?). A short-term stress that allows your mitochondria to adapt helps them become stronger. This means your cells produce more energy and you burn more fat, produce less toxins, and age gracefully. Fasting is one of the best hormetic stressors for your mitochondria.

Your thoughts have a huge influence on your aging process as well. As you'll learn later in the book, thoughts are frequencies that have the ability to penetrate your cell membranes and communicate with your DNA nucleus. If the thought is stressful or fearful, the signal sent is to produce inflammatory proteins. This shortens the telomeres around your DNA, which damages your DNA and ages you faster. If the thought is a positive and grateful thought, the signal sent to your DNA allows for anti-inflammatory proteins to be produced, lengthening your telomeres and protecting your DNA.[15, 16] Think about that for a second!

4. Reversing Autoimmune Conditions

When you think of autoimmune conditions, imagine a three-legged stool. If any leg of this stool is weak, the stool will lose its function by collapsing. Each leg of the stool needs to be addressed. With autoimmune diseases, the three legs of the stool are the gut microbiome, stressors, and genetic predisposition. We are going to address all three legs in this book.

We already discussed how fasting can reset your gut microbiome by giving it a break to repair itself through the process of energy diversion. Studies suggest that ketone bodies can significantly influence gut microbiota, offering potential benefits for reducing inflammation and improving metabolic and neurological health.

Genetics play a role in autoimmune conditions, but not as much as you think. There's growing research on the role of *epigenetics*, meaning "above the gene." It's true that you can't change the genes you were born with; however, you have the power to turn them on or off. The cell membrane and the mitochondria are the key players in this process.

We can absolutely heal our mitochondria and bring in the healthy fats to support cell membrane fluidity. This enables our cells to detox more efficiently, allowing nutrients and hormones into the cell and releasing free radicals outside of the cell. This is how epigenetics works. Our lifestyle influences genes that get turned on, and it also influences genes that get turned off.

I personally have two autoimmune conditions: Reynaud's syndrome and erythromelalgia. Raynaud's syndrome is a problem that causes decreased blood flow to the fingers. In some cases, it also causes less blood flow to the ears, toes, nipples, knees, or nose. This happens because of blood vessel spasms in those areas. Erythromelalgia, also known as Mitchell's disease, is a rare vascular disorder that causes pain, redness, and warmth in the extremities. The pain can be severe and burning, and the skin can become inflamed and hyperemic. Episodes can be constant or come and go, and they are often triggered by exercise or heat.

In 2018, I was visiting Seattle, Washington, with some friends, and we decided to take a day trip to a nearby alpine lake. We hiked for a couple of hours to get to one of the most beautiful scenes in nature I'd ever seen. The lake was fed directly by mountain snow, making the water extremely cold. I jumped in for a cold plunge for a couple of minutes. Upon exiting the water, I noticed my fingers were completely white. This was caused by the Raynaud's. The whiteness of my fingers traveled to my wrists as my body was diverting all its blood flow away from my extremities. This was a scary feeling because I couldn't even close my fist. I thought I was going to lose my fingers. I spent the next few minutes in a panic, looking for hikers who might be carrying a lighter. Thankfully, I found someone who gave me their lighter.

After 15 minutes of heating up my hands and fingers, the color returned to normal. This was an important lesson for me, as it showed me that I hadn't gotten to the cause of my Reynaud's syndrome yet. This is when I began to study the principle of hormesis. I was eating the right foods for my metabolism, but I hadn't addressed my toxicity load up until this point. I implemented the metabolic strategies outlined in this book and built up my hormetic ceiling. I'm happy to share that I rarely get Reynaud's symptoms these days. As a matter of fact, I own a cold plunge, and multiple times per week I find myself inside the plunge for three to four minutes at a time, without triggering any issues with my Reynaud's syndrome.

My other autoimmune condition is erythromelalgia. It's rare to have both Reynaud's and erythromelalgia because they both seem to oppose each other. Erythromelalgia would be triggered for me after eating a meal, especially a meal high in carbohydrates. My fingers would immediately turn red, hot, swollen, and inflamed. It would be so bad that I'd have to seek something cold to hold in my hands to alleviate the pain.

I fixed my gut microbiome with the ancient healing strategies and toxicity-reducing methods in this book. I'm happy to report that my erythromelalgia symptoms rarely occur now. I share these stories with you because it proves that your body can heal itself. You have the ability to turn off bad genes and turn on good ones. You are in control.

5. Detoxifying Your Body

Burning stored body fat for energy can move toxins out of your cells for excretion. Your body has a highly sophisticated system in place for toxins. When toxins enter, a pathway called PPAR-y gets turned on to shuttle the toxins out of your bloodstream and into your fat cells. Many of these toxins are lipophilic (fat-loving), and your fat cells are the perfect home for them. By shuttling toxins into your fat cells, it allows your body to mitigate the damage because the solution to pollution is dilution. As you'll learn later in this book, these toxins are called chemical obesogens because they increase fat cells, and your metabolism may recruit new fat cells to house these toxins. This process saves the body from harm in the short term while creating disease in the long term, unless it's addressed properly.

When you follow the steps outlined in your 30-day Metabolic Freedom Reset, you'll switch on fat burning, in which your metabolism burns stored energy (body fat) for fuel. When you practice intermittent fasting, it accelerates this process through autophagy, which is cellular cleanup. At this point all of your detox organs will move into action to ensure those toxins leave your system. Once you start using fat for energy, it mobilizes the toxins into your downstream detox pathways for removal. These detox pathways include your liver, kidneys, gut, gallbladder, and lymphatic system.

The more metabolic freedom you achieve, the more support these detox pathways will receive. Most people have closed detox pathways, which result in the following common symptoms:

- brain fog
- general and chronic fatigue
- constipation
- diarrhea
- skin abnormalities such as rashes
- feeling bloated after eating
- poor sleep

These symptoms are common, but they aren't normal. I've seen people who have tried every detox in the world overcome these symptoms with the 30-Day Metabolic Freedom Reset. You just need to work on opening up those downstream detox pathways, so that your body will effortlessly work on removing them without you even noticing. (In Chapter 5, I will show you specific protocols that work best for opening up your detox pathways.)

✦ ✦

Your metabolism doesn't have to slow down with age—it's a myth that aging alone causes a metabolic decline. The truth is, metabolic efficiency hinges more on lifestyle choices than on the passage of time. Muscle loss, reduced activity, poor nutrition, and chronic stress are the real culprits behind a sluggish metabolism. By prioritizing the tips outlined inside this book, and supporting metabolic flexibility through smart dietary choices, you can maintain a metabolism at age 70 that functions as efficiently as it did in your teenage years. Aging is inevitable, but a slowing metabolism is not. It's not just my opinion, recent scientific research challenges the common belief that metabolism inevitably slows with age. A comprehensive study published in *Science* analyzed data from over 6,600 individuals ranging from infancy to 95 years old. The findings revealed that, after accounting for body size and composition, total energy expenditure remains relatively stable from age 20 to 60—and even then, the changes are minimal after 60, with a gradual slowdown of approximately 0.7 percent per year.[17] I believe that even this modest slowdown can be prevented with the strategies in this book.

Now that you have a strong foundational understanding of the science of how your metabolism works, I'm excited to show you how to take these concepts and sync them with your hormonal needs. The following chapters will identify the main causes of metabolic dysfunction as well as the best ways to remove this interference and restore your metabolism for good. In the next chapter we'll examine the first cause: constant glucose and insulin spikes.

CHAPTER 3

BEING A
SUGAR BURNER

When I was a kid, I loved going to the arcade, and one of my favorite games was Whac-A-Mole. When you play Whac-A-Mole, you're given a toy hammer, and several holes in the play area in front of you are filled with small plastic cartoonish moles, or other characters, which pop up at random. Points are scored by, as the name suggests, whacking each mole as it appears. The faster the reaction, the higher the score. I was always going for the top score in my arcade!

Unfortunately, most people treat their health like a game of Whac-A-Mole. They experience a symptom popping up like a cartoon mole, and they use toy hammers such as medication, fad diets, surgery, and other extreme measures to whack it down. This might work in the interim, but you know what happens next: Another mole (symptom) shows up. In this never-ending world of symptom chasing, you'll find yourself exhausted with 23 hammers for 23 moles. In the game of life, the faster the reaction, the worse off you'll actually be.

As we discussed earlier in the book, your symptoms are not the same as your problems. In fact, most of the time symptoms are far removed from their causes. It isn't until you find out where the moles are coming from that you'll become successful at the game of your health.

Let's start with one of the peskiest moles to whack: constant glucose and insulin spikes.

Are You a Sugar Burner?

When your metabolism is stuck burning glucose, you become a sugar burner. Life is not fun for sugar burners—they create a lot of oxidative stress inside of their bodies, leading to a shortened health span and lifespan. In other words, if your goal is to age faster than anyone you know, burn sugar all the time.

I put together a six-question quiz to determine whether you're burning sugar or fat right now. If you answer yes to three or more of these questions, there's a high probability you're a sugar burner:

1. Do you feel tired after eating meals?
2. Do you snack in between your meals?
3. Do you have more than 20 pounds of extra weight on your body?
4. Do you have any skin tags on your body?
5. Do you have brown patches underneath your armpits?
6. If you skip a meal, do you get hangry (hungry and angry)?

If you scored as a sugar burner, it's not your fault; years of outdated information have led you down this path.

Your red blood cells keep a record of your blood sugar behavior. If you want to know for sure what's going on in your body, you can test your blood sugar levels by measuring hemoglobin A1C. Hemoglobin A1C (hbA1c) measures your average blood sugar from the past three months by detecting the glucose stuck to the hemoglobin protein. Your red blood cells carry oxygen to your tissues using a protein called hemoglobin A. The higher your blood glucose, the more glucose sticks to the hemoglobin A1C protein. A healthy hemoglobin A1C (hbA1c) is 5.2 percent or less, the prediabetic range is 5.7 to 6.4 percent, and the diabetic range is 6.5 percent or higher.

How glycated is your hemoglobin? Glycation is a spontaneous non-enzymatic reaction of free-reducing sugars with free amino groups of proteins, DNA, and lipids that form glycated residues. Sugar is sticky (think of cotton candy sticking to your fingers), and this sugar can gunk up your arteries and cells. The higher the A1C, the more glucose is glycated your protein.

A study from 2020 estimates that for both type 1 and type 2 diabetes, one year with HbA1c >7.5 percent loses around 100 life days. Linking glycemic control to mortality has the potential to focus minds on effective engagement with therapy and lifestyle recommendation adherence. I did the math for you: This means if your

HbA1c levels are >7.5 percent for 15 years, you lose 4 years off your lifespan.[1] The great news is that you are going to master your blood sugar levels and add years to your life!

When you're a sugar burner, there are five major ways it disrupts your metabolism:

1. chronically elevated levels of insulin

2. increased oxidative stress levels

3. depletion of your mitochondria

4. brain disorders

5. cancer growth

Let's dive in to each one of these now.

1. Chronically Elevated Levels of Insulin

Insulin is the body's main hormone switch. It determines which fuel you will use: fat or sugar. If insulin is high, no fat will be burned—only sugar. If insulin is low, fat will be used exclusively as fuel.

Insulin has a bad public relations person because it gets blamed for many things. But insulin production is actually a beautiful process that was designed by our creator; if we didn't have this process, humans wouldn't exist today. When we eat carbohydrates, our bodies convert them into sugar (glucose), which raises blood sugar levels. The body calls in the insulin troops to grab that sugar in the blood, and then insulin acts as a key to unlock your cells so that sugar can be moved into the trillions of cells.

If your blood sugar is normal, it means that you have roughly 1 teaspoon of dissolved sugar in your blood. An average person has about one gallon of blood in their body. So, you'd think that over the course of a day, you'd need very little sugar. But the average American consumes as much as 30 teaspoons of sugar every day! (This sugar typically comes from processed foods and carbohydrates.) Faced with this high amount of ingested sugar, the body needs to bring the blood back to homeostasis (its normal resting state), so anytime there's more than 1 teaspoon of sugar in the blood, insulin gets pumped into your blood to shuttle that glucose out of the blood and into your cells.

Just imagine how hard insulin must work to remove this massively excessive amount of sugar from the blood! It has to work *30 times* harder. That's insane.

The Lancet reported back in 2009 via the White Hall II study that fasting glucose remains unchanged for about 14 years; at this point the average person's pancreas has become fatigued from producing massive amounts of insulin over the years. The average doctor then diagnoses this person with diabetes, even though it has been developing for the last 14 years.[2] This is why the single most important lab test you can have to assess the health (or lack thereof) of your metabolism is a fasting insulin test. Albert Einstein said, "Intellectuals solve problems; geniuses prevent them," and it's a lot easier to work on preventing disease than trying to reverse it.

Elevated levels of insulin, hyperinsulinemia, evolve into type 2 diabetes. Conventional medicine treats the symptom (too much glucose), when the root cause is excessive insulin and cell membrane inflammation. By taking insulin, you are making the root cause and the type 2 diabetes worse. You can't superficially treat only the symptoms and expect the disease to get better. Insulin resistance (hyperinsulinemia) occurs years before diabetes. It's rare to die from diabetes, but many people die from the degenerative diseases connected to it: cancer, heart disease, infections, kidney failures, and so on. It all began with high levels of insulin. (In Chapter 12, you'll find that the 30-Day Metabolic Freedom Reset outlines the exact steps needed to lower insulin, so your cells can become sensitive to its messages.)

Your metabolism has a tightly controlled system for sugar in your bloodstream. Again, a healthy, thriving metabolism has only 1 teaspoon of sugar in the entire bloodstream. This equates to 80 mg/dL if you test your fasting blood sugar. Anything more is considered a toxic state.

We do have extra stores for sugar inside our liver and muscle cells called glycogen stores. On average, liver cells can store 25 to 30 teaspoons of sugar, and skeletal muscle cells can store about 100 teaspoons.

I love the analogy from my friend Dr. Jason Fung: Think of your glycogen stores (sugar reserves) as the refrigerator in your kitchen, and your stored body fat as the freezers in your basement. The benefit of using your refrigerator instead of a freezer is that it provides easy, quick access for food energy. You simply walk to your kitchen, open the fridge, and have available energy. The drawback is that it has limited storage capacity. You'd have to constantly put new groceries inside the fridge to maintain this balance. In other words, when you're burning stored sugar, you have to continually eat carbohydrates and snack every few hours to maintain energy; otherwise your stores decrease, and you crash.

The freezers in your basement are a smart choice because you can keep dozens of them full of energy. The drawback is that you'd have to wait a little longer to access the food inside any of those freezers, because it takes a few hours for the food to thaw before you can use it. In this example, the freezers represent your body fat. You might have hundreds of freezers' worth of energy, and a healthy metabolism flips the switch to start using this stored energy from body fat as a fuel source.

If you're like most people, though, you've continued to refill your glycogen stores in the refrigerator, never allowing a shift to burning stored body fat. When you consume 300 grams of carbohydrates or more per day, like the average American, and consume meals and snacks throughout the day, you are constantly raising glucose and insulin levels, keeping your metabolism burning sugar instead of fat. But don't worry—when we discuss ketosis and IF later in this book, you'll learn the most efficient way to tap into body fat for fuel.

2. Increased Oxidative Stress Levels

When cells rely solely on sugar for fuel, it creates oxidative stress and leads to weight gain, as sugar is an inefficient energy source. Burning sugar generates toxic by-products that cause inflammation around cells, disrupting hormone function and slowing metabolism. In contrast, fat is a cleaner, more efficient energy source, reducing cellular stress.

Phospholipase A2 (PLA2) is an enzyme that plays a crucial role in membrane lipid metabolism by hydrolyzing the sn-2 acyl bond of phospholipids, releasing free fatty acids and lysophospholipids. This enzyme is known to be involved in various cellular processes, including the inflammatory response and membrane remodeling. Think of PLA2 as a specialized pair of scissors for cell membranes. Just as scissors cut along a specific line, PLA2 snips the bond in membrane phospholipids at a precise spot, releasing free fatty acids and lysophospholipids. This "cutting" action is crucial for maintaining the balance and function of cell membranes, much like how trimming a plant helps it grow in a much healthier way.

Studies have indicated that spikes in sugar and insulin levels can influence the activity of PLA2, leading to potential membrane damage.[3] Imagine the cell membrane as a sturdy brick wall protecting a house. PLA2 acts like a demolition crew that removes specific bricks (phospholipids) from this wall. Normally, this process is controlled and helps with maintenance and remodeling. However, when sugar and insulin levels spike, it's like giving the demolition crew unchecked orders to remove bricks rapidly and randomly. This excessive activity weakens the wall, creating gaps and vulnerabilities. As a result, the house (cell) becomes more exposed to external threats and internal instability, leading to potential damage and dysfunction.

3. Depletion of Your Mitochondria

As discussed in Chapter 2, your mitochondria are the battery packs within your cells responsible for energy production and fat burning. Which car would you prefer, an old beat-up Ford Pinto or a brand-new Porsche, upgraded to the max? You'd want the Porsche, wouldn't you? Well, when you're in ketosis, your cells and mitochondria are that turbocharged Porsche.

Out of the trillion cells inside your body, you essentially have two main energy sources: sugar (glucose) and fat (ketones). When your body breaks down carbohydrates (sugar) for energy, it doesn't produce as much energy as when it breaks down fats. When your body breaks down fats for energy, it's like driving a sleek Porsche compared to burning sugar, which is more like driving a beat-up Pinto.[4, 5, 6, 7, 8]

In healthy humans, the body can easily produce ketones to be used for energy whenever it needs it. In times of fasting, and even overnight while sleeping on an empty stomach, the liver creates more ketones, and the amount of ketone bodies in the blood increases. When insulin is low enough, the body shifts into fat oxidation. These fatty acids are shuttled to the liver, and the liver uses them to produce ketones.

This means *keto is a metabolic process more than a diet*. Ketosis has been around for as long as humans have existed. If our ancestors couldn't use fatty acids for fuel and have the liver turn them into ketones, we wouldn't be here today! Our ancestors wouldn't have been able to focus enough to find food and would not have survived.

When you're using ketones instead of glucose, your mitochondria produce 400 percent more energy through mitochondrial biogenesis. This is because short-term ketosis is a beneficial stress (hormesis) on your mitochondria, which forces them to adapt and produce more energy. The result is an increase in heat inside your body, which raises your metabolic rate. When this is achieved, your metabolism burns more calories without having to count them, and without having to exercise excessively.

4. Brain Disorders

Recent research has begun to categorize Alzheimer's and Parkinson's diseases as "type 3 diabetes," highlighting a critical connection between insulin resistance and neurodegenerative disorders.[9] This emerging perspective suggests that just as type 2 diabetes is characterized by insulin resistance in the body, these brain disorders may stem from a similar resistance to insulin within the brain.

Insulin is essential not only for regulating blood sugar but also for neuronal health and function. When brain cells become resistant to insulin, it disrupts normal cellular processes, leading to cognitive decline and neurodegeneration. Understanding this link opens new avenues for treatment and prevention, emphasizing the importance of metabolic health in maintaining brain function and preventing these debilitating diseases.

In certain brain disorders, there can be a problem with transporting glucose into the neurons and/or other brain and nerve cells, and they essentially starve and die. Diseases/conditions with decreased glucose uptake into brain/nerve cells include:

- Alzheimer's disease
- Parkinson's disease
- multiple sclerosis
- Huntington's chorea
- ALS/Lou Gehrig's disease
- Duchenne muscular dystrophy
- some forms of autism
- Down syndrome (develop Alzheimer's disease by ages 30 to 40)[10]
- acute brain injury, accompanied by lack of oxygen
- type 1 and type 2 diabetes

Ketones can be taken up by neurons that cannot use glucose. Therefore, ketones may ameliorate the energy crisis in neurodegenerative diseases, which are characterized by a deterioration of the brain's glucose metabolism, providing a therapeutic advantage in these diseases. Most clinical studies examining the neuroprotective role of ketone bodies have been conducted in patients with Alzheimer's disease, where brain imaging studies support the notion of enhancing brain energy metabolism with ketones.[11] Likewise, a few studies show modest functional improvements in patients with Parkinson's disease and cognitive benefits in patients with—or at risk of—Alzheimer's disease after ketogenic interventions.

We've already established that ketones signal to the mitochondria to create more mitochondria by stressing them, and the brain has the highest concentration of mitochondria per cell than anywhere else in the body.[12] This is why so many people report clarity and mental resilience when they're in ketosis. This helps tremendously with the following conditions:

- Depression
- ADD
- ADHD
- Brain fog

The ketogenic diet helps with mood disorders by stabilizing blood sugar levels and reducing inflammation, which are key contributors to mood fluctuations. By shifting the body's primary fuel source from glucose to ketones, the brain receives a steady supply of energy, which can enhance mental clarity and emotional stability. Additionally, the keto diet promotes the production of gamma-aminobutyric acid (GABA), a neurotransmitter that has calming effects, potentially reducing symptoms of anxiety and depression. This metabolic shift can lead to improved mood regulation and overall mental well-being.[13, 14]

THE STATISTICS ON ALZHEIMER'S DISEASE

- In 2020, as many as 5.8 million Americans were living with Alzheimer's disease.

- Younger people may get Alzheimer's disease, but it's less common. Most people with Alzheimer's are age 65 and older.

- The number of people living with the disease doubles every five years beyond age 65.

- This number is projected to nearly triple to 14 million people by 2060.[15]

5. Cancer Growth

Research reveals that cancer cells heavily rely on glycolysis for energy, a phenomenon termed the Warburg effect.[16] Ketogenic diets present a promising avenue for cancer therapy by capitalizing on the metabolic vulnerabilities of cancer cells. According to the National Library of Medicine, keto works by starving tumors of their primary energy source—glucose—while providing alternative fuel for healthy cells.[17] By limiting carbohydrates and boosting ketone production, keto induces a metabolic state akin to fasting, effectively targeting cancer cells while preserving normal tissue. As succinctly stated by the National Library of Medicine, "Keto selectively starves tumors by providing the fat and protein that otherwise could not be used by glucose-dependent tumor cells."[18]

Keto further exerts its anti-cancer effects through various mechanisms, including inhibiting insulin/IGF pathways, prompting tumor cell death, and curbing tumor growth and spread. This comprehensive approach is bolstered by evidence showing keto's ability to alter gene expression, chromatin structure (controlling genetic expression), and crucial metabolic enzymes within tumor cells. Ongoing clinical trials further underscore the potential of keto in cancer treatment, aiming to validate its effectiveness and safety across different cancer types. In essence, by targeting the metabolic vulnerabilities of cancer cells, ketogenic diets offer a promising adjunct to conventional cancer therapies, potentially improving patient outcomes.

As you can see, there are a variety of dangers when you continue as a sugar burner. It's not just about feeling tired and gaining weight: the elevated insulin levels, increased oxidative stress, and diminished mitochondria place you at risk for neurogenerative diseases and cancer. Now that you have a solid understanding of how these high levels of glucose and insulin destroy your metabolism, let's discuss the next cause of metabolic dysfunction: processed foods.

CHAPTER 4

PROCESSED FOODS

Picture your average supermarket or drugstore: processed foods, made with ingredients most people can't pronounce, sit at the front of the store. The marketing of these foods is the best of the best, and people are easily enticed into buying them. Unfortunately, they also tend to develop health symptoms as a result of consuming these products, most commonly weight gain, headaches, heartburn, fatigue, and joint pain. Their doctors write a prescription for these symptoms, often sending them back to the same store, but this time to the pharmacy section to pick up the medication for the symptoms caused by eating the processed food. The healthcare industry turns symptoms into sales and diseases into dollars. It's a brilliant business model!

The sad truth is that a cured patient is a lost customer. I'm not a cynical person, but I am a realist. I know some amazing doctors truly care, but the healthcare system they are working in is broken. It's corrupt, it's not healthcare, and it's designed for sick care. Big Pharma has been selling us sickness for decades, and it's even reached a point where they are now creating sickness for us. This is because medication doesn't get to the root cause of why someone doesn't feel well, and often even makes that root cause worse.

We know we're heading in the wrong direction, and yet we struggle to find solutions. The issue isn't a lack of information; in fact, it's too much information. We're drowning in information but starving for true wisdom. Information alone will not change your life—if it did, every librarian would be a multimillionaire or celebrity. It's the application of the right information in a step-by-step system that will change your life. As you'll see in the pages ahead, despite the dire state we're in now, there's hope—but we need to make the right choices.

To achieve metabolic freedom, you must take sovereignty over your health information and the choices you make. If you treat your health casually, you will end up a casualty. In this chapter I'll strip the power away from Big Food, Big Pharma, and Big Gov, and give it back to you with the truth about processed foods and the real havoc they're wreaking on your body. Once you understand that the greatest physician and pharmacy you'll ever find is within your own body, you'll be able to take control over your health.

The Power—and Cost—of Marketing

Next time you watch TV, notice how many of the commercials are filled with pharmaceutical and food messages. I did some research and discovered that 75 percent of all television commercials in the United States are funded by Big Pharma![1] Out of the 195 countries in the world, only two of them allow Big Pharma to market directly to the consumer on television: the United States and New Zealand.[2] Big Food is all over television too, comprising up to 29 percent of advertisements![3] This means if you have the television on, you'll see medication after medication followed by fast food and more medication. This is intentional brainwashing of our conscious and subconscious minds—we don't have symptoms because of a lack of medication!

It gets worse. Why are fast food restaurants allowed to open shops inside hospitals? Hospitals should be a healing environment. It's corrupt, and it's designed to turn symptoms into sales and diseases into dollars.

The U.S. healthcare system ranked last overall among 11 high-income countries in an analysis by the nonprofit Commonwealth Fund.[4] Additionally, the United States spends 4.6 trillion dollars on healthcare every year. If this were a country's gross domestic product (GDP), it would be number four in the world!

Obesity is expensive, too. In 2008, the estimated annual medical cost of obesity in the United States was $147 billion, and the medical cost for people who have obesity was $1,429 higher than those of healthy weight.[5] *The Economic Report of the President*, which is published every five years, found that the total annual cost of diabetes in 2022 was $412.9 billion, including $306.6 billion in direct medical costs and $106.3 billion in indirect costs. People with diagnosed diabetes now account for one of every four healthcare dollars spent in the United States.[6] The average cost of treating a patient with type 2 diabetes is $14,000 per year.

Why is our (lack of) healthcare costing us so much? Why have the costs of obesity and diabetes skyrocketed? Because of the foods we are consuming.

How Processed Foods Damage Metabolic Health

Our supermarkets and convenience stores are riddled with processed junk food. If I smoked a cigarette in public, most people would think *dude, smoking kills*, yet if I consumed processed junk food loaded with sugar, they wouldn't have a second thought about it. But processed foods kill more people than cigarettes, and there's a drug dealer on every corner. Human beings are the only species smart enough to create their own food and dumb enough to eat it.

A 2024 meta-analysis revealed that a diet high in ultra-processed foods showed some alarming statistics. Ultra-processed foods are heavily altered with additives and unhealthy ingredients, posing greater risks to metabolic health than minimally processed foods, which retain more of their natural nutrients. This study showed that ultra-processed food may increase the following:

- diabetes by 37 percent
- high blood pressure by 32 percent
- high triglycerides by 47 percent
- obesity by 32 percent[7]

Such "foods" are destroying our metabolic health. They negatively impact our metabolism in five key ways:

1. They are highly addictive.
2. They create cellular inflammation.
3. They cause mitochondrial damage.
4. They signal fat storage.
5. They disrupt the gut microbiome.

Let's look at each of these in detail.

1. They Are Highly Addictive

The food scientists working behind the scenes for big food companies are brilliant. They manufacture these food-like substances called frankenfoods and test them several times to ensure they hit all the reward centers in your brain. Take Doritos, for example: The premise behind Doritos Roulette is that the bag contains a mix of regular Nacho Cheese Doritos and a few extremely spicy chips, which are indistinguishable from the regular ones. These spicy chips measure about 78,000 Scoville heat units, making them significantly hotter than a typical jalapeño. This unpredictability adds a thrill to the snacking experience, as consumers never know when they might encounter one of the fiery chips.[8]

Recent research has highlighted the startling similarities between sugar and addictive drugs like cocaine. Studies conducted on rats have shown that sugar can be more addictive than opioid drugs. These studies found that sugar triggers responses in the brain comparable to drugs, including binging, craving, tolerance, withdrawal, dependence, and reward.[9]

Dr. James DiNicolantonio, the lead author of a review published in the *British Journal of Sports Medicine,* explains that sugar affects the brain's dopamine levels, leading to symptoms like depression and ADHD when consumption is suddenly reduced. This dopamine deficiency can drive the urge to consume more sugar, similar to the "fix" that drug addicts seek.

Unlike salt, which has a natural aversion signal preventing overconsumption, sugar lacks such a mechanism, allowing people to consume large amounts without feeling the need to stop. This continuous consumption can lead to various metabolic health issues, including weight gain, heart disease, type 2 diabetes, stroke, and some cancers.

The research also points out that while the addictive behaviors seen in rats might not directly translate to humans, the high sugar intake, especially among children, is a cause for concern. Public Health England reports that sugar intake in the United Kingdom is nearly three times the recommended limit, contributing significantly to the overall energy intake.[10] Sugar is processed in a way that causes overconsumption, since it does not activate the hormone leptin, which signals to your body and brain to put down the fork.

2. They Create Cellular Inflammation

An estimated 80 percent of the food supply in the United States contains inflammatory seed oils. These oils are also called vegetable oils, linoleic acid, polyunsaturated fats, and omega-6 fats. The main problem with these fats is that they are chemically unstable. They contain many double bonds, which is where the term "poly" comes from, and the more double bonds a fat contains, the more unstable it is to heat and pressure. When food companies manufacture and process these oils, they add heat and pressure, which damages these fats, making them rancid. They cover up the rancid look and smell with chemical agents that include hexane, phosphoric acid, bleaching agents, steam, and others.

This means seed oils sitting on the shelf are already rancid before you even purchase them. When you heat them during cooking, these fats oxidize further. This creates cellular inflammation, blocking the hormones and nutrients from entering your cells. It's similar to the oxidation that occurs after you've bitten into an apple and left it on the counter for hours. The browning is oxidation, and these oils create this "browning" at the cell level.

3. They Cause Mitochondrial Damage

Health experts disagree about many things, but if there's one thing we can all agree on it's this: Healthy mitochondria are essential for metabolic health. When your mitochondria are healthy, your cells produce energy so that you thrive throughout the entire day, and this burns fat by raising your metabolic rate. Processed foods, however, are essentially mitochondrial poison.

Many of these processed foods contain high amounts of high fructose corn syrup (HFCS), which raises uric acid levels inside the body. This is a metabolic disaster, as elevated uric acid levels are linked to an increased risk of developing dementia and Alzheimer's disease. Additionally, uric acid directly contributes to insulin resistance, further complicating metabolic health.

Our bodies tend to retain uric acid as an evolutionary survival mechanism, a trait inherited from our primate ancestors. Historically, higher uric acid levels helped conserve fat stores for periods of scarcity. In modern times, this mechanism has become outdated, as we do not hibernate or face prolonged food shortages. This retention can now be detrimental, because individuals with elevated uric acid levels are also at a higher risk of severe outcomes from illnesses such as COVID-19.

The human body can process a limited amount of fructose, approximately 5 grams at a time. Consuming fructose in higher amounts, especially from sources like fruit juice, can overwhelm the body's metabolic capacity. Excessive fructose consumption is a primary contributor to gout, a painful condition characterized by high uric acid levels. In his book *Nature Wants Us to Be Fat*, Dr. Richard Johnson explains that animals in the wild consume large quantities of fruit before hibernation to gain fat. In humans, however, such dietary patterns can lead to the accumulation of fat in the liver, resulting in insulin resistance, diabetes, and increasing the risk of cancer and heart disease.

By understanding and managing uric acid and fructose intake, we can make significant strides in improving metabolic health and preventing related diseases. Consuming HFCS and rancid seed oils is like pouring sand into the engine of a finely tuned car. It leads to an increase in uric acid, which acts like grit, causing oxidative stress and inflammation. This stress hampers the mitochondria—the cell's power plants—from running efficiently, reducing their ability to produce energy (ATP) and disrupting overall cellular metabolism. Over time, this "engine trouble" can lead to bigger issues like obesity, insulin resistance, and other metabolic disorders, underscoring the importance of a clean diet in keeping our cellular engines running smoothly and preventing chronic disease.

4. They Signal Fat Storage

As we established, the two primary causes of weight gain and weight-loss resistance are cellular membrane inflammation and high levels of insulin. Processed foods are a metabolic nightmare because they create both of these problems. Processed carbohydrates, such as cereals, cookies, bread, and others, spike insulin after consuming them, which signals to your body to "store fat." The artificial ingredients found in processed foods inflame cell membranes, making your hormones work harder to do their job of burning fat and producing energy.

Over time, hormones must work harder, leading to hormone resistance, as the inflammatory levels of a cell continue to increase. This increases the risk of obesity, weight gain, and weight-loss resistance.

5. They Disrupt the Gut Microbiome

Hippocrates nailed it a long time ago when he said, "All disease begins in the gut." Fast-forward to 2020, and Harvard published a study titled "All disease begins in the (leaky) gut: role of zonulin-mediated gut permeability in the pathogenesis of some chronic inflammatory diseases" by Alessio Fasano.[11] In this study, Fasano explores the role of gut permeability, specifically through the protein zonulin, in chronic inflammatory diseases. The research highlights how increased intestinal permeability, often termed "leaky gut," allows toxins and antigens to enter the bloodstream, triggering inflammatory responses. The study underscores the importance of maintaining gut barrier integrity for overall health.

Processed foods disrupt the lining of your digestive system by creating inflammation and leaky gut. Leaky gut, or increased intestinal permeability, occurs when the tight junctions in the gut lining become loose, allowing harmful substances like toxins, microbes, and undigested food particles to pass into the bloodstream. This can trigger inflammation and immune responses, contributing to various health issues, such as autoimmune diseases, chronic inflammatory conditions, digestive disorders, metabolic disorders, and brain fog, since the gut is connected to the brain via the vagus nerve. Factors such as poor diet, stress, infections, and certain medications can contribute to the development of leaky gut, highlighting the importance of maintaining a healthy gut barrier for overall well-being.

When you become aware of the hidden junk food that surrounds you, you can make better decisions that will serve your future self. Neville Goddard once said, "We are only limited by weakness of attention and poverty of imagination." We do the best we can according to our level of awareness. This is why it's important to become aware of the environment that surrounds you, which includes television commercials, billboards, your social media feed, and even your friends and family.

Now that you're aware of the prevalence of processed foods and their dangerous effect on metabolic health, let's dive into the next cause of metabolic dysfunction: environmental toxins.

CHAPTER 5

ENVIRONMENTAL TOXINS MAKE YOU SICK AND INFLAMED

We live in a toxic world. The Environmental Working Group (EWG) examined the cord blood of newborns and found that they began life exposed to as many as 287 of the 413 toxic chemicals featured in the study.[1] Of the chemicals found, 180 are known to cause cancer. Cancer rates in children have also risen 67.1 percent since 1950. According to the Columbia University School of Public Health, "95 percent of cancer is caused by diet and the environment."[2]

Toxic chemicals have been linked to severe health issues, including cancer, birth defects, and other chronic diseases, affecting both the environment and local communities. Environmental toxins are everywhere—we can find them in the pesticides on our food, in our cleaning supplies, in our beauty products, and more. We need more rigorous environmental regulations to protect public health from these pervasive and dangerous toxins.

Scientists are still researching the way the environment impacts our hormones from substances like BPA (bisphenol A), which is a chemical used in plastics and resins that can disrupt hormones and may negatively impact health when leached into food and drinks, and flame retardants in fabrics, furniture, curtains, and carpets. However, we do know that many of the chemicals in our environment are endocrine disruptors that interfere with our hormones and wreak metabolic havoc on our bodies. But it's not all doom and gloom.

The good news is that your body is equipped with natural detoxification systems designed to eliminate harmful toxins. Later in this chapter, I'll share specific protocols to help you activate and support these detox pathways. But before we dive into that, let's first explore where these toxins originate.

Where Are We Getting This Toxic Load?

Environmental toxins are abundant. They are in cleaning supplies, cosmetics, personal care products, shower curtains, amalgam fillings in teeth, the water and food supply, and, yes, even the air freshener your Uber driver blasts you with as you enter the vehicle. Studies have found that individual cash register receipts can contain BPA that is 250 to 1,000 times greater than the amount in a can of food.[3] Just say no when a salesperson asks if you want a receipt at a store.

Then there are microplastics: A University of Newcastle study, which was commissioned by the World Wildlife Fund, found that the average person consumes around 2,000 tiny pieces of plastic each week, or about 5 grams, which equates to the weight of the average credit card.[4] A groundbreaking study published in March 2024 in the *New England Journal of Medicine* revealed a significant link between microplastics in arterial plaque and an increased risk of heart attacks, strokes, and mortality. The study analyzed plaque samples from 304 patients undergoing carotid endarterectomy, a procedure to clear blocked arteries. Microplastics were found in 58.4 percent of the patients' plaque, primarily polyethylene and polyvinyl chloride. Over a follow-up period of two to three years, those with microplastics in their plaque were approximately 4.5 times more likely to experience severe cardiovascular events or death, underscoring the potential dangers of microplastic exposure.[5]

TIPS FOR REDUCING YOUR PLASTIC CONSUMPTION

To reduce your ingestion of microplastics:

- Drink out of glass bottles instead of plastic ones.
- Don't heat up plastic Tupperware in the microwave, or better yet, replace them with glass storage containers.
- Switch from plastic cutting boards to wooden cutting boards.
- Be sure to rinse your dishes and dry them before you use them, as there is a significant amount of plastic from our household environment that accumulates on our dishes while they sit in our kitchen cabinets.

Glyphosate

If you've ever been to Europe, you'll notice a vast difference in the health of the locals versus the tourists from the United States. Take Italy, for example—studies show that only 12 percent of people who live in Italy are obese. Compare this to the United States, where close to 50 percent of people are obese.[6] Diabetes in Italy is also a fraction of what we see in the United States, at a rate of only 5.3 percent, compared to the United States, which is more than double.[7] The life expectancy in Italy is 82.8 years, compared to 76.3 years in the United States.[8, 9] Is it because more people work out in Italy than the United States? Not exactly—there's a fraction of the gyms in Italy compared to the United States. The difference is that Italy and many other European countries have banned toxins like glyphosate from the food supply.[10]

Glyphosate is a broad-spectrum herbicide commonly used to kill weeds, particularly in agricultural settings, and it works by inhibiting a specific enzyme pathway necessary for plant growth. Concerns have been raised about its potential effects on human health, particularly regarding its impact on metabolism. Some studies suggest that glyphosate may disrupt gut microbiota, impairing digestive health and leading to metabolic disorders. Additionally, it has been linked to potential endocrine disruption, which can interfere with hormonal balance and contribute to metabolic diseases like obesity and diabetes.[11]

Data published by MIT researcher Stephanie Seneff and Anthony Samsel shows strong correlations between the application of glyphosate on the U.S. food supply and specific diseases and conditions like dementia, diabetes, autism, Alzheimer's, and Parkinson's. Their research highlights how the widespread application of this herbicide closely aligns with the growth of these serious health issues over time.[12] Furthermore, in her book *Toxic Legacy: How the Weedkiller Glyphosate Is Destroying Our Health and the Environment*, Seneff shares research on glyphosate's ability to push heavy metals, such as mercury, lead, aluminum, and others, deep inside of our tissues. Glyphosate opens up the blood-brain barrier, allowing toxins to enter the brain, which bioaccumulate during their lifetime. It's estimated that glyphosate is in at least 60 percent of our rainfall![13]

Glyphosate removes vitamins and minerals from your body, starving your cells and not allowing your mitochondria to produce energy and burn fat, creating metabolic dysfunction. The most common crops sprayed with glyphosate include coffee, wine, beer, corn, soy, and wheat. This is why I suggest the following:

- Choose organic, non-GMO foods as much as possible.

- Look up the "Clean Fifteen" and the "Dirty Dozen." The "Clean Fifteen" are fruits and vegetables with the lowest pesticide residues, while the "Dirty Dozen" are those with the highest, as identified by the Environmental Working Group (EWG) to help consumers make safer produce choices.

- Take high-quality fulvic and humic minerals to remove glyphosate. Fulvic and humic acids are natural compounds found in soil that support nutrient absorption, gut health, and detoxification by binding to and removing toxins and delivering minerals to cells.

- Keep your detox pathways open (more on this shortly).

- Move to Italy!

Endocrine Disruptors

Chemicals in the environment, known as endocrine disruptors, can affect the body's endocrine system by mimicking naturally occurring hormones. In response, the body may over- or under-produce the mimicked hormones and others. Endocrine disruptors have been linked with developmental, reproductive, brain, immune, and other problems.

Even low doses of endocrine-disrupting chemicals may be unsafe. The body's normal endocrine functioning involves slight changes in hormone levels, and we know that even these small changes can cause significant developmental and biological effects.

These disruptors are commonly found in everyday products like plastics (BPA), personal care items (phthalates), pesticides, and industrial chemicals (PCBs). PCBs are toxic, man-made chemicals that were once used industrially but are now banned due to their environmental persistence and health risks. To avoid them, it's best to choose products labeled as BPA-free, use glass or stainless-steel containers instead of plastic, opt for organic produce to reduce pesticide exposure, and select natural or fragrance-free personal care products. Additionally, filtering your water and minimizing processed foods can help reduce exposure to these harmful chemicals.

Toxic Obesogens

The old "calories in versus calories out" model for weight loss doesn't account for the role of environmental toxins. According to a study found in the *Journal of Diabetes Investigation*, new risk factors for obesity and diabetes are environmental chemicals.[14] They are calling these toxins obesogens because of the impact they have on the obesity crisis we face. A study from *Environmental Health Perspectives* made a strong connection between toxins and weight gain. They cite that many in the medical and exercise physiology communities remain wedded to poor diet and lack of exercise as the sole cause of obesity. However, researchers are gathering convincing evidence of chemical "obesogens"—dietary, pharmaceutical, and industrial compounds that may alter metabolic processes and predispose some people to gain weight.[15]

Worldwide obesity has more than doubled since 1980, and if current trends continue, 50 percent of adults in the United States will be obese by 2030. Adding to this problem is an increasing amount of evidence suggesting that endocrine-disrupting chemicals (EDCs) may also play a role. Two terms have been coined to describe the role of certain chemicals in metabolism and obesity:

1. **Obesogens** are chemicals that can enter the body and disrupt normal lipid metabolism, which can lead to obesity.

2. **Diabetogens** are chemicals that can enter the body and kill B cells or disrupt their function and interfere with normal energy metabolism, which can lead to diabetes.[16]

The body stores lipophilic "fat-loving" chemicals in our fat as a survival mechanism to prevent them from freely circulating in the body.[17] Current obesity reports state that "it is noteworthy that obesogen structures are mainly lipophilic, their ability to increase fat deposition has the added consequence of increasing the capacity for their own retention."[18] This toxic load has the potential for a vicious spiral not only of increasing obesity but also of increasing the retention of other lipophilic pollutant chemicals with an even broader range of adverse actions. Our high toxic load might offer an explanation as to why obesity is an underlying risk factor for so many diseases, including cancer.

The potential for a "vicious spiral" to be set up where obesogens act to increase the amount of fat stored (be it by increased cell volume or increased cell number) would be followed by greater retention of lipophilic obesogens, which would then lead onward in an increasing spiral of greater body fat and even more lipophilic pollutant retention. In this sense, obesogens may be self-fulfilling and able to increase capacity for their own retention.[19]

HOW TOXINS CAUSE WEIGHT GAIN

- They increase the number of fat cells.
- They increase the size of fat cells.
- They alter basal metabolic rate.
- They alter the hormones regulating appetite and satiety.
- They alter endocrine regulation of adipose (body fat) tissue.
- They alter energy balance in favor of storing calories.
- They alter insulin sensitivity and fat metabolism in endocrine tissues.

Heavy metals, which include lead, mercury, aluminum, arsenic, and cadmium, are what I call super toxins. They can accumulate in the body, leading to chronic health issues and weight gain. These metals can create inflammation by generating oxidative stress, which damages cells and tissues, disrupts normal cellular functions, and triggers the immune system to respond. Over time, this chronic inflammation can contribute to a range of diseases, including cardiovascular problems, neurological disorders, and autoimmune conditions. Common sources of heavy metal exposure include contaminated water, silver amalgam fillings, certain foods (like fish high in mercury), industrial pollution, lead-based paints, and some household products. To reduce exposure, it's important to filter drinking water, choose low-mercury fish (the smaller the fish, the fewer the toxins), avoid products with known heavy metal contamination, and be cautious of environmental pollutants.

Simple Ways to Open Your Downstream Detox Pathways

Your body has natural detoxification pathways designed to eliminate toxins. The 30-Day Metabolic Freedom Reset in Chapter 12 is specifically crafted to help activate and enhance these pathways. Here are some simple strategies to further support your body's detox processes:

- Sweat regularly.

- Pursue an active lifestyle.

- Incorporate bitter-rich foods into your diet (we'll dive into this more later).

- Apply a castor oil pack around your liver.

- Consider coffee enemas.

- Engage in lymphatic drainage techniques.

These practices will help ensure your detox pathways are functioning optimally.

Once you start your reset, your detox pathways will open up to assist you in eliminating these accumulated toxins. When this happens, your stress bucket is reduced, and you'll feel better.

In the next chapter we'll examine the final problem causing metabolic dysfunction: lack of adequate sleep.

CHAPTER 6

LACK OF QUALITY SLEEP

Sleep is like the master switch for metabolism: When you improve your sleep, every aspect of your metabolism improves; but when your sleep suffers, your entire metabolic system struggles.

Personally, lack of quality sleep impacts me more than any other poor lifestyle behaviors. Quality sleep may be more important than nutrition and exercise combined. That's a bold statement, but I know the following to be true: I can go days without food or exercise and be just fine, but if I went days without sleep, I'd turn into a hallucinating metabolic nightmare. Sleep builds the foundation of health, and without it, the foundation will be weak. Your health will fall apart, brick by brick. Prioritizing quality sleep will supercharge every aspect of your metabolism.

My client Sandy was desperate to lose weight. He became 90 pounds overweight, developed prediabetes and high blood pressure, and relied on a sleep apnea machine each night. Sandy has a wife and teenage daughter, and he was worried about setting a bad example for them and not being around long enough to see his daughter grow up. During our first conversation, I had him share his routine with me. I discovered that he was waking up early to go to the gym before work every day. He was sacrificing sleep to exercise. I explained to Sandy that exercise is fantastic, but sleep is foundational. Exercise is something we add in once the foundations are stable. I encouraged him to stop waking up early to hit the gym and instead get those two extra hours of sleep.

Just four weeks in, Sandy was down 14 pounds by getting more sleep. He had more energy for work and family, and eventually once this sleep foundation was solid, we slowly brought in exercise. Fast-forward to today, and he's lost 70 pounds.

He no longer relies on his sleep apnea machine, and the best part, he inspired his wife, Margaret, to follow a similar lifestyle, and she went on to lose 35 pounds.

Unfortunately, many of us, like Sandy, aren't getting enough sleep. This can disrupt our metabolic health in a number or ways, including increased insulin levels and a buildup of toxins, which we'll explore in this chapter. I'll also reveal the habits that wreck your sleep the most, so that you can be sure to avoid them and practice good sleep hygiene.

The Stats on Sleep

Sleep deprivation is an alarming issue in the United States, with about 35 percent of adults not getting the recommended seven hours of sleep each night.[1] This pervasive lack of sleep has been recognized as a public health crisis by the Centers for Disease Control and Prevention (CDC). The average American now sleeps only about 6.8 hours per night, a significant decline from previous decades, reflecting a disturbing trend toward chronic sleep insufficiency.[2]

The repercussions of this widespread sleep deprivation are profound, affecting millions of Americans. Between 50 and 70 million adults suffer from sleep disorders, with insomnia being the most prevalent.[3] Approximately 30 percent of adults experience insomnia, and 10 percent face chronic insomnia that severely impacts their daily functioning.[4] This issue has far-reaching consequences for both individual health and public safety.[5]

Encouraging better sleep habits and prioritizing sufficient rest can lead to significant benefits, including enhanced physical health, improved mental clarity, and greater overall life satisfaction.[6] As the statistics make clear, ensuring adequate sleep is a fundamental component of a healthy lifestyle, essential for maintaining optimal metabolic health and well-being.[7,8]

Lack of Sleep = Metabolic Dysfunction

The health implications of inadequate sleep are extensive. Sleep deprivation is linked to an increased risk of obesity, diabetes, cardiovascular diseases, and various mental health disorders. The strain on the body from lack of rest exacerbates these conditions, leading to a cycle of poor health outcomes. Moreover, sleep deprivation significantly impacts safety, contributing to nearly 20 percent of all car accidents, highlighting its role in many preventable injuries and fatalities.[9]

Lack of sleep contributes to metabolic dysfunction in the following four key ways:

1. increased blood glucose and insulin levels
2. slowed metabolism
3. toxicity buildup leading to brain disorders
4. circadian rhythm mismatch

Let's look at each of them in turn.

1. Increased Blood Glucose and Insulin Levels

Imagine your body as a well-orchestrated symphony, where each instrument represents a different aspect of your metabolism. Sleep acts as the conductor, ensuring that each instrument plays its part harmoniously. When you don't get enough sleep, it's as if the conductor is absent, causing the orchestra to fall out of sync. The stress hormones (like cortisol) start playing too loudly, drowning out the soft, steady rhythm of insulin, which is crucial for regulating blood sugar. Simultaneously, the hunger hormones (ghrelin and leptin) start playing erratic and conflicting tunes, leading to overeating. This chaos results in a disjointed performance in which blood sugar levels rise uncontrollably, much like a symphony gone awry without its conductor.

In one study, the authors found that after one week of shortened sleep, your blood sugar levels are disrupted so significantly that your doctor would classify you as being prediabetic. When you're not getting quality sleep, the beta cells in your pancreas stop being sensitive to the signal of high glucose.[10] Research presented at the Experimental Biology 2009 meeting highlights the link between short or poor sleep and increased risk of overeating and type 2 diabetes. Studies, such as those published in the *Annals of Internal Medicine* and the *Journal of Clinical Endocrinology & Metabolism*, and others, highlight how sleep restriction in healthy adults results in decreased insulin sensitivity and hormonal changes that increase appetite and calorie intake.[11, 12, 13] These studies show that sleep deprivation disrupts appetite regulation, leading to overeating and higher insulin resistance. Stress responses and hormonal changes, including elevated stress hormones and reduced insulin, further complicate the relationship between sleep, eating behaviors, and diabetes risk.

A study published in *Diabetes* found that restricting sleep to five hours per night for one week significantly reduces insulin sensitivity in healthy men. The study involved 20 healthy participants and demonstrated a 20 percent reduction in insulin sensitivity following sleep restriction. This reduction was associated with increased cortisol levels but not affected by the alertness drug modafinil. The findings highlight the adverse effects of short-term sleep deprivation on glucose metabolism, raising concerns about the potential long-term impacts on insulin resistance and related metabolic disorders.[14]

Poor sleep elevates cortisol levels, which leads to the destruction of collagen in the skin, muscle breakdown, and bone degradation. This process supplies amino acids to the liver for glucose production, resulting in higher blood glucose levels. Consequently, this can cause insulin resistance, as the body overproduces glucose, prompting the pancreas to release insulin. Caffeine, often consumed to counteract sleep deprivation, can exacerbate cortisol production. Cortisol directly affects cells and indirectly prompts the liver to release glucose, making cells insulin resistant even without glucose changes, as observed in cell cultures treated with cortisol-like molecules.[15, 16, 17]

If you drink caffeinated beverages, it's a good idea to wait at least 90 minutes after waking to consume them. Waiting 90 minutes has several benefits: It allows your body to naturally decrease cortisol levels, which are typically high upon waking. Consuming caffeine too early can further elevate cortisol, leading to increased stress and anxiety. By delaying caffeine intake, you help maintain a more balanced cortisol rhythm, enhancing alertness naturally. Additionally, this practice can prevent the midday energy crash often associated with early caffeine consumption, promoting sustained energy levels throughout the day.

2. Slowed Metabolism

Research shows that a lack of sleep can significantly slow down your metabolism, much like a car engine running inefficiently without proper maintenance. Sleep deprivation disrupts the balance of hormones related to hunger and appetite, decreasing leptin (which suppresses appetite) and increasing ghrelin (which stimulates appetite). This hormonal imbalance can lead to increased food intake and weight gain. Additionally, as we just discussed, sleep deprivation reduces insulin sensitivity, making it harder for the body to process glucose efficiently, which can result in higher blood sugar levels and an increased risk of type 2 diabetes. Inadequate sleep can lower the resting metabolic rate (RMR), which means the body burns fewer calories at rest, contributing to weight gain.

Elevated levels of cortisol (the stress hormone) due to lack of sleep, can be compared to a car's engine overheating, causing more stress on the system. High cortisol levels can lead to increased appetite and fat storage, especially in the abdominal area. Studies have shown that individuals who sleep less tend to have higher levels of body fat. The reduction in sleep often results in fatigue and a lack of motivation to engage in physical activity, further decreasing overall energy expenditure.[18] Ensuring adequate sleep is thus crucial for maintaining a healthy metabolism and preventing metabolic disorders.

Growth hormone plays a critical role in regulating metabolism, body composition, and overall health. It's essential for stimulating growth, cell reproduction, and cell regeneration. Growth hormone promotes the synthesis of protein, which is vital for muscle growth and repair. It also increases the breakdown of fats into free fatty acids, which can be used as an energy source, thus helping to reduce body fat. Growth hormone supports the maintenance of normal blood glucose levels by reducing the uptake of glucose in tissues and enhancing glucose production in the liver. During deep sleep, also known as slow-wave sleep, growth hormone secretion is at its peak. This stage of sleep is crucial for the body's recovery and repair processes. When individuals do not get enough deep sleep, the production of growth hormone is significantly impaired. This deficiency can interfere with various metabolic processes. For instance, inadequate growth hormone levels can lead to decreased muscle mass and increased fat accumulation. It can also impair the body's ability to regulate blood glucose levels, increasing the risk of insulin resistance and type 2 diabetes.

Lack of deep sleep can therefore disrupt the delicate balance of metabolism. Without sufficient growth hormone, the metabolism becomes inefficient, and the body's ability to burn fat and build muscle is compromised. This can lead to weight gain and a higher proportion of body fat. Additionally, the impaired glucose regulation associated with reduced growth hormone can exacerbate metabolic issues, further contributing to the risk of metabolic disorders. Ensuring adequate deep sleep is therefore vital for maintaining optimal growth hormone levels and supporting a healthy metabolism.

3. Toxicity Buildup Leading to Brain Disorders

In his book *Why We Sleep,* Dr. Matthew Walker delves into the intricate workings of the glymphatic system, emphasizing its crucial role during sleep. The glymphatic system, a waste clearance system in the brain, becomes highly active during deep sleep. It functions similarly to the lymphatic system in the rest of the body, clearing out metabolic waste products accumulated during the day. Dr. Walker explains that during sleep, especially in the deeper stages, cerebrospinal fluid flows more freely through the brain tissue, effectively removing toxins such as beta-amyloid, which is associated with Alzheimer's disease.

Walker highlights that the efficiency of the glymphatic system during sleep underscores the importance of adequate sleep for maintaining brain health. When we do not get enough sleep, the brain's ability to clear out these toxins is compromised, leading to a buildup that can contribute to neurodegenerative diseases. His research points to the alarming fact that chronic sleep deprivation may increase the risk of developing Alzheimer's disease and other cognitive impairments due to the insufficient removal of these harmful substances.

Walker's work emphasizes that sleep quality, not just quantity, is vital for the optimal functioning of the glymphatic system. Deep, non-REM sleep is particularly important, as it is during this phase that the glymphatic system operates most efficiently. Ensuring good sleep hygiene and prioritizing deep sleep can significantly impact overall brain health, reducing the risk of cognitive decline and supporting long-term mental well-being. Walker's research in *Why We Sleep* provides compelling evidence that sleep is not merely a passive state but a dynamic process essential for maintaining brain health and preventing neurodegenerative diseases.

4. Circadian Rhythm Mismatch

Research strongly indicates that lack of sleep and night shift work are associated with an increased risk of various health issues, including cancer and a shortened lifespan. The World Health Organization's International Agency for Research on Cancer (IARC) has classified night shift work as a probable carcinogen, primarily due to its disruption of the circadian rhythm.[19] Circadian rhythms regulate vital physiological processes, including sleep-wake cycles, hormone release, and metabolism. Disruption of these rhythms, common among night shift workers, can lead to hormonal imbalances and impaired cellular function. Studies have shown that this disruption can increase the risk of several types of cancer, including breast, prostate, and colorectal.

The increased cancer risk among night shift workers is attributed to several mechanisms. One key factor is the suppression of melatonin, a hormone produced at night that regulates sleep and has antioxidant properties. Exposure to light at night suppresses melatonin, leading to increased oxidative stress and DNA damage, which promotes cancer development. Additionally, disrupted sleep impairs the immune system, making it less effective at detecting and destroying cancer cells. These findings highlight the critical role of maintaining regular sleep patterns and minimizing circadian disruption to mitigate cancer risk.

In addition to the increased cancer risk, lack of sleep and night shift work are associated with a shortened lifespan. Chronic sleep deprivation and circadian misalignment contribute to metabolic and cardiovascular issues, including obesity, diabetes, hypertension, and heart disease. A study published in the journal *SLEEP* found that individuals with irregular sleep patterns had a higher risk of mortality from all causes compared to those with regular sleep patterns.[20] The cumulative effects of sleep deprivation and circadian disruption can accelerate the aging process, leading to earlier onset of age-related diseases and ultimately shortening lifespan.

The Worst Lifestyle Habits That Wreck Your Sleep

Now that you understand the importance of quality sleep as it relates to metabolic health, let's discuss some of the worst behaviors that lead to poor sleep. The first poor behavior is eating too close to bedtime. When you give your metabolism energy in the form of food and proceed not to use it because you lie down for bed, your metabolism is signaled to store every bit of that energy. Eating food raises your body temperature, which is the opposite of what you want to do before sleep. To enter deep sleep, our body temperature needs to drop by about 1 to 2 degrees Fahrenheit (approximately 0.5 to 1 degree Celsius). This drop in temperature signals to the body that it's time to transition into the deeper stages of sleep, where restorative processes occur. The cooling down process helps facilitate the onset of sleep and maintains the optimal conditions for deep, restful sleep.

Eating before bed is like throwing a surprise party for your stomach just when it's trying to wind down for the night. Imagine you've just settled into your comfy bed after a long day, ready to drift off to sleep, and suddenly, a group of friends bursts into your room, ready to party. Your peaceful night is disrupted, and instead of relaxing, you're now wide-awake and dealing with the commotion. Similarly, when you eat right before bed, your digestive system gets a wake-up call just when it should be slowing down. The process of digestion kicks into high gear, making it harder for your body to relax and enter the deep, restorative stages of sleep. This can lead to indigestion, acid reflux, and disrupted sleep patterns, turning what should be a restful night into a restless one. Just like you wouldn't throw a party when it's time to sleep, it's best to avoid eating large meals right before bed to ensure a peaceful night's rest. I recommend no food at least three hours before bedtime.

The next bad habit is eating against your natural circadian rhythm. Circadian rhythms are the natural, internal processes that regulate the sleep-wake cycle and repeat roughly every 24 hours. These rhythms are driven by the body's biological clocks, which are present in nearly every cell and synchronized by a master clock in the brain known as the suprachiasmatic nucleus (SCN). The SCN is located in the hypothalamus and responds primarily to light and dark signals, which help regulate various physiological processes, including hormone production, metabolism, and sleep.

Imagine your body as a quirky, bustling amusement park called "Circadian Land." This park runs on a strict schedule set by a whimsical clock tower, the central timekeeper. This clock tower represents the brain's suprachiasmatic nucleus (SCN), which keeps everything in sync, from the roller coasters to the snack stands. In Circadian Land, hormones are like the park's energetic staff members. Cortisol, the park's perky morning greeter, gets everyone pumped up and ready for a day of fun. Melatonin, the night guard, gently ushers everyone out when the park closes, ensuring things are quiet and restful for the night.

When the park follows its schedule, the rides operate smoothly, the food stands serve tasty treats on time, and everyone has a great day. But if the park's schedule gets messed up—imagine the roller coasters running at 3 A.M. and the snack stands serving breakfast at midnight—chaos ensues. The staff gets confused, rides break down, and guests start feeling queasy. This is what happens when our circadian rhythms are disrupted by irregular sleep or eating patterns. Hormonal imbalances occur, leading to metabolic issues, weight gain, and even mood swings.[21, 22]

To keep Circadian Land running like a dream, it's essential to stick to a regular schedule. Time-restricted eating is like having fixed park hours, ensuring the rides (your metabolism) and staff (hormones) work in harmony. This helps maintain balance and promotes overall health, much like a well-timed amusement park providing endless fun and joy to its visitors.[23, 24]

Dr. Sachin Panda, a prominent researcher in the field of circadian biology, has significantly advanced our understanding of how the body's internal clock influences health and well-being. In his groundbreaking book, *The Circadian Code,* Dr. Panda explores the intricate relationship between our biological rhythms and daily habits, particularly our eating patterns.[25] His research reveals that the timing of our meals can profoundly impact metabolism, weight management, and overall health. By aligning our eating schedules with our natural circadian rhythms, we can optimize bodily functions, improve energy levels, and reduce the risk of chronic diseases.

Dr. Panda's work emphasizes that our bodies are designed to follow a 24-hour cycle, with specific times for activity, rest, and nourishment. Disrupting this cycle through irregular eating habits, such as late-night snacking or skipping meals, can lead to metabolic imbalances and health issues. Dr. Panda advocates for time-restricted eating, wherein food intake is confined to a specific window of time each day. This approach not only synchronizes our internal clocks but also enhances metabolic efficiency, supports weight loss, and lowers the likelihood of developing conditions like diabetes and heart disease. By adopting eating patterns that honor our circadian rhythms, we can harness the power of our biological clock to achieve optimal health and vitality.

Dr. Panda's research has provided substantial insights into how the timing of food intake can affect metabolic health. One pivotal study demonstrated that mice given access to food around the clock became obese and developed various metabolic diseases, including high cholesterol, fatty liver, and diabetes. In contrast, mice that consumed the same high-fat diet but were restricted to a feeding window of 8 to 10 hours remained lean and healthy. This striking difference was attributed to better alignment with their circadian rhythms, which regulate gene expression, hormone levels, and other metabolic processes.[26, 27]

Incorporating Dr. Panda's insights into our daily routines can lead to transformative changes in our health. His research underscores the importance of not just *what* we eat, but *when* we eat. By embracing a lifestyle that respects our circadian rhythms, we align ourselves with the natural order of our bodies, promoting a harmonious balance that fosters long-term well-being. As we strive for better health, understanding and implementing the principles of circadian biology can serve as a crucial foundation for achieving lasting metabolic health and overall wellness.

Sleep is the key to unlocking your metabolic freedom. Make sure your foundation is rock solid, and everything else in this book will work that much better. Now that we've explored the primary causes of metabolic disease, let's dive into the most effective solutions for restoring your metabolic health.

In Part II we'll look at some of the solutions to these problems, starting with why keto is so valuable for metabolic health.

THE
SOLUTIONS

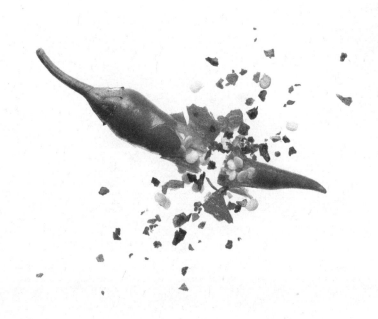

CHAPTER 7

WHY KETO IS THE ANSWER TO METABOLIC FREEDOM

If there's one word that strikes a combination of dread and cynicism in the hearts of overweight people, it's the word *diet*. So let's clear up one bit of misinformation here: *Keto is not a diet—it's a metabolic process.* It's nothing new; it's just nuanced. Its origins are deep in human history, as every single one of our ancestors did keto. Burning fat and using ketones is our primal birthright.

Every cell inside of your body is hardwired to use this metabolic process of fat burning from time to time. Did you know that soon after babies are born, they enter a natural state of ketosis? Yep, you read that right—research shows that newborn infants are in ketosis and remain in this normal, healthy state while breastfeeding. Furthermore, research confirms that breast milk from healthy mothers is actually made up of 50 to 60 percent fat, *and* the cholesterol in breast milk supplies babies with almost six times the amount that most adults consume in their diets.[1] Keto-adapted babies can efficiently turn ketone bodies into acetyl-coA and myelin, which helps the development of the baby's brain since it is made mostly of fat.

As we know, the body can burn only two types of fuel: fat and sugar. Earlier in the book, I referenced a study showing that 93 percent of U.S. adults are metabolically unhealthy, and I'm going to make the case that it's because of a keto deficiency! The first step to metabolic freedom is teaching your body how to burn fat again.

In Chapter 3, we identified whether you are a sugar burner or a fat burner, and now we're going to teach your cells to switch fuel sources from sugar (glucose) to fat (ketones). In this chapter I'll share some of the extraordinary benefits of ketones, which foods to avoid as well as the best ones to add to your diet, and how to support your liver during this process.

Ketones Can Turn Genes On and Off

As we established in previous chapters, epigenetics run the show: Ketones, or the state of ketosis, have been shown to turn off bad genes that were turned on from poor lifestyle behaviors.

In ancient times, our ancestors were forced into ketosis during times of famine or limited carbohydrates (such as the winter). This means that keto has been around since the dawn of humankind. I would go as far as to say that we wouldn't exist today if it wasn't for the metabolic process of ketosis. When our ancestors did not have food, they fasted. This fast could have been for only hours, but sometimes it lasted days to weeks. As glucose dropped inside the body and the brain, a metabolic switch to fat and ketones was made. This fueled our ancestors' brains and bodies so they could remain sharp, focused, and energized to hunt and kill their next meal. If it wasn't for this metabolic switch to burning fat and ketones, our ancestors would have been blubbering idiots with low energy—they wouldn't have been capable of finding food, and they would have gone extinct.

You've likely heard the phrase "survival of the fittest." In this context, "fittest" refers to those who can activate genes that promote longevity and deactivate genes linked to disease by harnessing the power of ketones.

THE 6 KEY BENEFITS OF KETONES

- increase cellular energy via mitogenesis
- reduce inflammation and its markers
- elevate growth hormone and protection of all cells and DNA from oxidative stress
- increase ATP production (cellular energy)
- burn cleaner metabolically than glucose (fewer free radicals)
- protect and repair the inner mitochondrial membrane

The Mechanisms of Action for Ketosis

The mechanisms of action for ketosis encompass a wide range of beneficial effects on metabolic health. Ketosis lowers blood sugar and insulin levels, while ketone bodies act as important signaling molecules that trigger a cascade of effects throughout the body. These include anti-seizure properties, alterations in neurotransmitter systems—such as increased levels of GABA and adenosine and decreased glutamate—and changes in ion channel regulation. Ion channel regulation is the process of controlling the movement of ions across cell membranes, which is essential for cellular functions like signaling, muscle contraction, and maintaining the body's balance of fluids and electrolytes.

Ketosis also enhances mitochondrial function and production, reduces inflammation by upregulating antioxidants like glutathione peroxidase and lowering inflammatory cytokines, and decreases leptin levels. Additionally, ketosis positively impacts the gut microbiome, influences DNA methylation and gene expression, increases autophagy, boosts NAD+ levels (NAD+ levels reflect a vital molecule for energy and cell repair, declining with age), and activates sirtuin genes (sirtuin genes regulate aging, cell repair, and metabolism), all of which contribute to improved cellular health and longevity.

Ketosis Improves Many Health Conditions

Research has shown that ketosis can play a significant role in managing and improving several chronic and complex diseases. Polycystic ovary syndrome (PCOS) is one such condition where ketosis has demonstrated benefits. Studies indicate that a ketogenic diet can help regulate insulin levels, which are often elevated in PCOS, thereby improving symptoms and fertility outcomes.[2] Acne, another common condition, may improve with ketosis due to its effects on reducing insulin levels and inflammation, both of which are implicated in the pathogenesis of acne. Similarly, obesity and hyperlipidemia, both major risk factors for cardiovascular disease, have been effectively managed through ketosis. By promoting fat loss and improving lipid profiles, ketosis offers a compelling approach to weight management and metabolic health.

Epilepsy, particularly drug-resistant forms, has long been treated with ketogenic diets, with numerous studies validating its anti-seizure effects.[3] This approach has been so effective that it's considered a gold standard treatment for epilepsy in both children and adults. Moreover, neurodegenerative diseases like Alzheimer's and

Parkinson's disease may benefit from ketosis, as ketones provide an alternative energy source for brain cells, potentially slowing disease progression and improving cognitive function.[4, 5] Autism spectrum disorders may also benefit from a ketogenic diet, with preliminary research suggesting improvements in behavior and cognition.[6]

Emerging research also suggests that ketosis might play a role in cancer therapy. Some studies propose that because many cancer cells rely heavily on glucose, a ketogenic diet, which lowers blood sugar, might slow tumor growth.

In the realm of metabolic diseases, ketosis has shown promise in managing diabetes by improving insulin sensitivity and glycemic control. Additionally, ketosis has been linked to improvements in cardiovascular health, reducing high blood pressure, and ameliorating conditions like fatty liver disease by decreasing liver fat and improving overall liver function.

Foods to Avoid During Ketosis

When you conduct a quick search on "Dr. Google" for the keto diet, it will provide you with over 200 million results! It's enough information to confuse the heck out of you. One thing's for sure: There's not one way to do it. Many people who supposedly teach keto do not do so with respect to the body at the cellular level. Yes, there are certain foods that will get you into ketosis, but will they actually help you achieve perfect health? In this section we'll cover the foods you definitely want to avoid, such as inflammatory fats and artificial ingredients.

Inflammatory Seed Oils (a.k.a. Vegetable Oil)

One of the most important nuggets of keto research I've encountered over the years has been about bad fats. They're considered bad because they're unstable, rancid fats that wreak cellular havoc inside the body. (See Chapter 4.) I remember sitting down for a *Metabolic Freedom* podcast interview with MIT research professor Brian Peskin, where I asked him about these bastardized fats. I asked him which he believed was worse for our health, these unstable fats or smoking cigarettes. Given his analytical mind, he said, "Let's look at the research." It turns out that if someone smoked two packs of cigarettes every day for 28 years, their chance of developing lung cancer within those 28 years is 16 percent. Compare that to someone consuming cooked vegetable oils every day for 28 years. Their chance of developing cancer and/or heart disease is 86 percent. Yikes!

When I later interviewed Dr. Cate Shanahan, M.D., author of *Deep Nutrition* and *Dark Calories*, on my podcast, I asked if her research aligned with Professor Peskin's. She said that when you consume these industrial seed oils it raises your risk of disease closer to 100 percent! During this same interview, I presented Dr. Shanahan with three scenarios that lead to disease:

1. smoking cigarettes daily
2. eating processed sugar daily
3. consuming vegetable oils daily

I asked her which scenario will create disease faster inside of the body. She chuckled and said, "Easy question, Ben. It's the vegetable oils."

Dr. Martin Grootveld estimates that in the average 5-ounce serving of fries, "aldehyde contents are not dissimilar to those arising from the smoking of a [daily] allocation of 25 tobacco cigarettes." A large order of McDonald's fries contains 20 to 25 fries. For each French fry you eat, you can imagine that you just smoked a single cigarette.[7] Aldehydes can cause cancer by damaging DNA and proteins, leading to mutations and cellular dysfunction.

These unstable fats offer no value to the body. When they're consumed, they gunk up your cell membranes and integral membrane proteins (receptor sites), which leads to an increase of inflammation. Dietary fatty acids incorporate into your cell membranes within hours after consuming them through a process called lipid membrane reorganization. Yes, you really are what you eat, and it happens a lot faster than most people think. When rancid fats embed into your cell membranes and mitochondrial membranes, they block the communication from your hormones, nutrients, and oxygen. When you have cellular membrane inflammation, toxins can't get out of the cell and nutrients and hormones can't get in. This eventually leads to disease, which first shows up as a symptom.

In addition, cell membrane inflammation remains long after the inflammatory vegetable oils have been removed. Studies suggest that the half-life of linoleic acid (omega-6 fats) is 680 days! Meaning, if you removed these bad fats from your diet today, 680 days later, about half of them will still be in your body fat creating problems.

Imagine a childhood friend who shows up to your house uninvited. He enters your house and plops himself on your couch, eats your food, makes a mess in your bathroom, and doesn't leave for 680 days! This is what you're doing to your cells each time you eat these unstable fats. Yes, these fats may help you enter "ketosis," but they will lead to a destructive path.

It's important to note that not all omega-6 fats (seed oils) are bad for you—it's the processed, adulterated versions of these fats that make them highly inflammatory. Most of the time, these oils are the adulterated version. If you can find unadulterated versions of seed oils, such as organic, cold-pressed sunflower, safflower, or grapeseed oil, they can help protect your cell membranes—provided they are not heated.

It's estimated that 80 percent of the food supply in the United States contains inflammatory seed oils.[8] It's a shame the American Heart Association puts their stamp of approval on these oils, stating they are "heart healthy," when in reality they are the complete opposite.

The harmful oils you want to avoid are:

- canola oil (also called rapeseed oil)
- corn oil
- soybean oil
- cottonseed oil
- rice bran oil
- sunflower oil
- refined peanut oil
- fish oil
- grapeseed oil
- refined palm oil
- hydrogenated oil
- safflower oil

Obesogens

You also want to avoid a group of foods filled with chemicals that create inflammation inside your body, which ultimately will make your keto experience really hard. As we discussed in Chapter 5, these chemicals are often referred to as *obesogens*. Many of them can spike both glucose and insulin and can stimulate the hunger centers in your brain, which makes the keto lifestyle more difficult to sustain. They are in many popular health products, such as cereals, flavored yogurts, protein bars, low-calorie snacks, sugar-free beverages, and light salad dressings, so make sure you read the labels.

Common synthetic ingredients to avoid:

- acesulfame potassium
- aspartame
- sucralose
- saccharine
- NutraSweet
- red or blue dyes
- artificial colors and flavorings

How Many Carbohydrates Can You Have on Keto?

I don't advise avoiding carbs altogether or adding more of them, so they don't really fall into the "foods to avoid" or "foods to add" sections. In general, most people can achieve ketosis by dropping their total carbohydrates to 50 grams per day. Others might need to be more restrictive, usually those who have been sugar burners for a long time. I don't recommend dropping your carbohydrates below 50 total grams too soon; instead, I suggest a gradual approach. When you aggressively lower your carbohydrates, it can lead to symptoms such as weakness, fatigue, and headaches, causing people to quit keto.

As you'll see in Chapter 12, I've outlined the exact steps for you to achieve a fat-burning state in less than a week. Most of your carbohydrate intake should come from non-starchy vegetables like broccoli, arugula, cauliflower, mushrooms, Brussels sprouts, zucchini, and asparagus. These nutrient-rich vegetables provide healthy carbohydrates that won't cause a significant spike in glucose, helping you stay in fat-burning ketosis.

Foods to Add

As you begin to remove some of the harmful foods that you've been consuming throughout your lifetime, you may be wondering what to replace them with. The goal is to prevent unwanted symptoms, such as cravings. The best way to stop these cravings is to stabilize your blood sugar and subdue your hunger hormone ghrelin.

This can be accomplished by following the gradual decrease in carbohydrates, which will be outlined for you in your 30-Day Metabolic Freedom Reset, and by adding more good fats and protein to your diet.

Healthy proteins to add:

- grass-fed and finished beef and lamb (i.e., raised on a natural grass diet for their entire lives, resulting in higher levels of beneficial nutrients like omega-3s and antioxidants)
- pasture-raised turkey and chicken
- bison
- pasture-raised pork
- pasture-raised eggs
- charcuterie meats like salami and prosciutto (nitrate free)
- sardines
- salmon
- anchovies
- herring
- mackerel

The best fats for cooking at high temps:

- grass-fed butter
- grass-fed ghee
- beef tallow
- duck fat
- coconut oil
- lard (non-hydrogenated from pastured pigs)

The best fats for salad dressings, dips, and low-heat cooking:

- avocado oil
- extra virgin olive oil

Approved alternative sweeteners:

- erythritol
- xylitol
- Swerve
- pure stevia
- monk fruit
- allulose

Support Your Liver

The liver is the "MVP" organ, because it completes so many important tasks for the human body, especially when it comes to detoxification and fat loss. After taking over 5,000 people through a keto protocol, I discovered the number one reason why people fail to achieve success on keto: a sluggish, backed-up liver.

Many people have a sluggish liver from medications, toxins, processed foods, and/or alcohol. One of the liver's roles is to produce bile acids (also called bile salts or hepatic biliary sludge). Bile is a fluid that is made and released by the liver and stored in the gallbladder. Along with bile acids, it contains water, cholesterol, bilirubin (a breakdown product of old, recycled red blood cells), and other trace elements, and it helps to break down fat-soluble vitamins (A, D, E, and K). When you start to increase healthy fats but fail to break them down properly, digestive distress occurs. The most common symptoms are loose stools and diarrhea. Thick, biliary sludge also leads to fatigue, since the process of bile production and secretion by the liver, known as choleresis, is a metabolically active process that requires a ton of energy. Not to mention, a significant amount of the sugar your body has stored over the years is housed in your liver, primarily in the form of glycogen. The liver plays a key role in regulating blood sugar levels by storing and releasing glucose as needed, especially during fasting, intense exercise, or between meals. When we consume high-sugar foods, any excess glucose not immediately used for energy is stored in the liver. Over time, these reserves can build up, leading to an overburdened liver, which may contribute to metabolic dysfunction. Reducing stored sugar allows the liver to operate more efficiently, which benefits blood sugar stability, fat metabolism, and overall metabolic health.

Imagine your liver as a factory that never stops working, constantly producing a special detergent called bile. This detergent is essential for breaking down fats in your diet, much like how a dishwasher detergent breaks down grease on dishes. Even when the kitchen is closed and no meals are being served, this factory keeps churning out detergent to be ready for the next meal. Now, if the production line slows down and the detergent piles up, the factory must use extra energy to manage and recycle the leftover detergent. This energy comes from the factory's power source, ATP, which is also used for other important tasks like burning fat. So, when the factory diverts its energy to handle the excess detergent, it has less power available to keep the fat-burning processes running efficiently.

Sluggish bile production can drain your metabolic energy, impacting your overall metabolism and ability to burn fat. Harvard Medical School researchers have explored the relationship between bile acids and metabolic health. Studies from the Department of Molecular Metabolism at Harvard indicate that bile acids play a critical role in regulating metabolism by influencing gut microbiota and immune function. For example, bile acids can activate specific signaling pathways that improve metabolic processes and reduce inflammation, potentially leading to better overall metabolic health.[9]

A study conducted at Tampere University Hospital in Finland found that people with decreased bile flow are seven times more likely to experience hypothyroidism. This connection is believed to be due to the role of bile in the conversion of thyroid hormones. Specifically, bile helps trigger the release of an enzyme that converts the inactive thyroid hormone T4 into its active form, T3. This process is crucial for maintaining proper thyroid function. Additionally, gut bacteria involved in bile metabolism also play a role in this hormonal conversion, further linking bile health to thyroid function.[10,11]

Research also suggests that poor bile production and flow may be linked to chronic fatigue and chronic fatigue syndrome (CFS), as well as migraines. In fact, studies have indicated that there is a higher prevalence of migraines among individuals with CFS, with symptoms often exacerbated by chronic fatigue and systemic pain.[12, 13] Additionally, gut inflammation, which can be influenced by bile production, has been identified as a significant factor in CFS. Altered gut microbiota and increased gut permeability, resulting in higher levels of inflammatory markers, have been observed in CFS patients.[14]

Consume Bitter Foods for the Liver

The solution is bitter foods, so let's take a moment to discuss them now. Ever wonder why coffee is so popular? Here's one reason: It's one of the few truly bitter foods remaining in the typical American diet, and it's also one of the few foods rich in antioxidants. In fact, research has revealed that coffee provides up to 45 percent of the antioxidants in typical Western diets.[15] Even though coffee is a small percentage of our total food and beverage consumption, because it's so rich in antioxidants, which is also what makes it bitter, it can account for a large percentage of our antioxidant intake.

These bitter antioxidants provide a wealth of health benefits, especially when they're eaten in keto-friendly foods as part of your regular diet. Research has shown that they reduce inflammation, improve blood sugar control and insulin sensitivity, increase metabolism in fat cells, and reduce blood pressure. They also support your gut microbiome and may even help protect against cancer.[16]

You can dampen the bitter flavor of many vegetables while keeping the health benefits by leveraging fat to make delicious recipes. The great chef Julia Child, who had no tolerance for fake foods, said, "With enough butter, anything is good." Her love of butter went against the mainstream attitude. Many "experts" preached that butter led to heart attacks. As usual, Julia Child was ahead of her time. She also reportedly said, "If you don't like broccoli, put more butter on it."

Bitter foods—including many herbs, leafy greens, ginger, lemons, limes, apple cider vinegar, cacao, and bitter melon—all contain fat-soluble vitamins as well as liver-boosting nutrients such as sulfur. These are necessary for the body to be able to produce bile, which, as I mentioned before, is needed for optimal digestion and to help the liver work at prime level. It breaks down fats into fatty acids, which can be taken into the body by the digestive tract.

For thousands of years, people have used "bitters" as digestive tonics. These have typically included leaves, roots, or flowers in an alcohol base, which are imbided after a large meal. There may be solid science to support these beliefs. That's largely because bitters may trigger the production of stomach acid, which facilitates a variety of digestive processes when the food you've eaten makes its way to the intestinal region. Additionally, bitters may increase the production of digestive enzymes, which further aids food absorption.

Bitter foods to support the liver in breaking down fat:

- arugula
- organic coffee
- apple cider vinegar
- lemons/limes
- radicchio
- rosemary (dried or fresh)
- thyme (dried or fresh)
- basil (dried or fresh)
- dill (dried or fresh)
- ginger and ginger tea
- milk thistle tea
- Brussels sprouts
- broccoli
- dandelion greens
- Jerusalem artichokes
- saffron
- sesame seeds
- turmeric
- grapefruit
- peppermint
- green tea

Once you are fat-adapted through ketosis, the next step is to add intermittent fasting into your lifestyle. Keto and fasting pair perfectly together like bacon and eggs. They are both ancient healing strategies that have been around since humankind. In the next chapter, we'll explore the incredible metabolic benefits of fasting.

CHAPTER 8

THE FASTING FIX FOR TAPPING INTO STORED BODY FAT

When people think of fasting, the image that often comes to mind is a skinny guy wearing a simple robe, sitting cross-legged in a monastery on a mountaintop. It has a decidedly spiritual context, in which the cleansing of the body is connected to the cleansing of the soul. In such a context, fasting is not connected to "real life," in which you must go to work, get the kids off to school, clean the house, and complete all the mundane tasks we do every day.

In this book, we look at fasting differently. Responsible, smart fasting is meant for everyday life. It plays an integral role in your daily health and well-being, and therefore you need to know as much as you can about it. I believe fasting is nature's reset button. There are many different ways to practice it, from daily intermittent fasting to extended water fasts—the key is to follow a schedule that keeps you within your hormetic zone, as we've discussed. Think of fasting like using a chainsaw. If you take the time to read the user manual before using it, you'll see great results with this powerful tool. But if you skip the manual and try to use a chainsaw without any knowledge, you could easily hurt yourself. The tool is important, but how it's wielded is just as crucial.

As you begin your 30-Day Metabolic Freedom Reset, I'll guide you through IF protocols, starting with 12-hour fasts to build that muscle. We'll gradually work our way to longer fasts, ensuring that you stay within your hormetic zone for optimal success. I understand that the idea of fasting, especially if you've never tried it before, may seem as daunting as holding your breath for five minutes. However, the way you'll be practicing it will feel manageable, because you've already made the effort to strengthen your metabolic machinery.

In this chapter I'll share the latest research on the benefits of fasting, which include lowering blood pressure, digestive health, brain health, and metabolism efficiency.

The Remarkable Benefits of Fasting

Back in 2014, I began researching the benefits of fasting. I was so excited to learn about this ancient healing tool that I immediately applied it to my schedule and experienced incredible results. I remember posting on my Facebook page about intermittent fasting, and I received so many concerned messages: "Ben, you are starving yourself. You are encouraging an eating disorder. You are going to wreck your metabolism." I didn't expect so much pushback! Back then the research was more limited, but now we have plenty of evidence showing how effective fasting can be. *Fasting* has even become one of the top search terms on Google.

One of the most comprehensive and highlighted studies ever conducted on the subject was published in *The New England Journal of Medicine* in December 2019. The authors reviewed more than 85 studies and suggested that IF should be used as the first line of treatment for diabetes, obesity, cancer, neurodegenerative brain conditions, and cardiovascular disease. The study examined an 18:6 IF method, which involves fasting for 18 hours each day followed by a 6-hour eating window. The study also revealed that IF has anti-aging benefits. This meta-analysis highlighted several key cellular healing benefits, including:

- increased antioxidant defenses
- increased cellular repair via autophagy
- increased ketones
- increased mitochondrial stress resistance
- increased DNA repair
- decreased glycogen
- decreased protein synthesis
- decreased mTor
- decreased insulin

In terms of what we're covering in this book, fasting will achieve four key benefits when it comes to restoring your metabolism:

- lowering high blood pressure
- digestive health
- brain health
- metabolism efficiency

Let's take a closer look at each of these.

1. Lowering High Blood Pressure

An estimated 103 million American adults have high blood pressure, according to recent statistics from the American Heart Association.[1] That's nearly half of all adults in the United States. The death rate from high blood pressure increased by nearly 11 percent in the United States between 2005 and 2015, and the actual number of deaths rose by almost 38 percent—up to nearly 79,000 by 2015, according to the statistics.[2] "Worldwide, high blood pressure affects nearly a third of the adult population and is the most common cause of cardiovascular disease-related deaths," said Paul Muntner, a professor and vice chair in the Department of Epidemiology at the University of Alabama at Birmingham.

According to the National Kidney Foundation and American Heart Association, high blood pressure cannot be cured, but it can be managed with medication. Is this true?

Throughout the 20th century, scientists noticed that when they took away food from patients with high blood pressure, their blood pressure levels would begin to drop. As the days passed, the pressure continued dropping until it eventually reached normal levels and flattened out. This was seen in a 1915 study of prolonged fasting from the Carnegie Institution, where patients underwent prolonged fasting for varying lengths of time, with some fasting for as long as 31 days.[3]

In the 1990s, Alan Goldhamer began to study the effects of fasting on a large group of individuals. Goldhamer runs the TrueNorth Health Center in Northern California, the largest medically supervised water-only fasting clinic. They looked at 174 of Goldhamer's patients who came to TrueNorth with high blood pressure. They fasted on average for a week and a half on nothing but water and found that 154 (nearly 9 out of 10) normalized their blood pressure.[4]

Goldhamer and his colleagues submitted his groundbreaking findings to 30 journals, and they were rejected each time. Why would the medical community be interested in a healing tool that is free? There are billions of dollars to be lost from Big Pharma and Big Food if people catch on to the healing benefits of fasting.

A fun fact is that airline pilots visit Goldhamer's TrueNorth clinic once a year to perform a 10-day water fast, so they can keep their blood pressure optimal, which is required to fly an airplane. If you're concerned that I might ask you to go without food for days, don't worry. The 30-Day Metabolic Freedom Reset is designed to help you achieve similar results with shorter fasting schedules. Think of it like tuning a car engine—you don't need to overhaul the entire engine to improve performance; sometimes, just removing a few blockages can make it run smoothly. Similarly, by allowing your metabolism to function more efficiently and eliminating any interference, you'll see the benefits without needing to endure extended fasts.

2. Digestive Health

We usually think of food as giving us energy, but digesting the food we eat actually *requires* energy, as we discussed in Chapter 2. After a heavy meal, an estimated 65 percent of the body's energy must be directed to the digestive organs. Chewing food and allowing the body to take macronutrients and assimilate them into micronutrients for distribution is a big task. During fasting, we rest our system from the constant onslaught of food and redirect our energy toward healing and recuperation. Our body can detox, repair cells, and eliminate foreign toxins and natural metabolic wastes.

Imagine a corporate employee named Jennifer who works 9:00 A.M. to 5:00 P.M. each day, putting in a full day of work. She clocks out of her job after a long day and walks to her car. As she approaches her vehicle, thinking about going home to rest and recover, she receives a phone call from her boss asking her to return to the office to work on an important project for the next five hours. Reluctantly, she goes back and puts in the extra work. It is now 10:00 P.M., and Jennifer is exhausted and ready to go home and rest. As she approaches her car again, she receives another phone call from her boss asking her to come back to the office to work on another project.

Imagine this happening to Jennifer for days, and even weeks, on end—she would begin to lose her ability to function. This is exactly what you're doing to your digestive system when you're not practicing IF. From the perspective of the gut, you're not giving it the time it needs to rest in between meals.

After every meal, there is a little bit of endotoxemia (meaning the presence of endotoxins in the blood). Endotoxins are toxic substances, primarily made up of lipopolysaccharides (LPS), that are found in the outer membrane of certain bacteria in the gut. After eating a meal, these endotoxins can be released into the bloodstream if the gut barrier is compromised. This release can trigger an inflammatory response in the body, as the immune system reacts to what it perceives as a threat. Over time, repeated exposure to endotoxins can contribute to chronic inflammation and various metabolic disorders. It can vary by the types of foods and fats that you're eating, and it can be worsened if you have a leaky gut. When you *don't* eat, you reduce that endotoxemia, so you're allowing the body to do its cleanup work to reduce inflammation and rebalance itself.

If you look historically at the number of meals that people ate 50 years ago compared to now, it used to be only three meals a day, and now it's five or six meals per day. If this is the case with you, you're not giving your body enough time for your blood sugar and insulin levels to drop, and the internal balance that improves your sensitivity to insulin can't occur. When you're eating too many meals, you're not allowing that rest period that's necessary for the body to be able to hit the reset button in between. We were not meant to live with a continuous influx of calories!

One meal can create an energy expenditure from the body for up to 72 hours, and that can take 70 to 80 percent of your energy levels. Think about that. I'm talking about the Standard American Diet, which is indeed SAD. We are overwhelming the digestive system, and it cannot keep up with the demand.

Fasting gives your digestive system a break, so it can use its resources for healing. I have seen this work well for the following digestive symptoms:

- acid reflux
- gas
- bloating
- puffiness
- GERD
- diarrhea
- leaky gut
- autoimmune conditions

My client Patricia had been battling fatigue and brain fog for years. Despite trying various extreme diets, many of which encouraged frequent snacking between meals, she found herself feeling worse rather than better. Her energy levels were consistently low, her mind felt clouded, and she struggled with persistent digestive issues, particularly acid reflux. It seemed that no matter what she tried, nothing could shake the constant feeling of exhaustion and mental sluggishness.

When Patricia learned about fasting and we began to slowly build up her fasting muscle, everything changed. By gradually extending the time between meals, we allowed her metabolism to reset and function more efficiently. Patricia now reports having the energy of a teenager, with her brain firing on all cylinders. Her once-debilitating brain fog has lifted, and her digestive issues, including the persistent acid reflux, have completely disappeared. This is why I call fasting nature's reset button!

Regenerating Intestinal Stem Cells

Stem cells are special human cells that can develop into many different cell types, ranging from brain cells to muscle cells. In some cases, they can also fix damaged tissues. You might say that stem cells are the body's ubiquitous, all-purpose cells from which all other cells with specialized functions are generated.

As you get older, your intestinal stem cells begin to lose their ability to regenerate. Because these stem cells are the source for all new intestinal cells, this decline can make it more difficult for an aging person to recover from gastrointestinal infections or other conditions that affect the intestine.

According to research from MIT biologists, this age-related loss of stem cell function could be reversed by a 24-hour fast.[5] The researchers found that fasting dramatically improves stem cells' ability to regenerate, in both aged and young mice.

"Fasting has many effects in the intestine, which include boosting regeneration as well as potential uses in any type of ailment that impinges on the intestine, such as infections or cancers," said Omer Yilmaz, an MIT assistant professor of biology, a member of the Koch Institute for Integrative Cancer Research, and one of the senior authors of the study.

"This study provided evidence that fasting induces a metabolic switch in the intestinal stem cells, from utilizing carbohydrates to burning fat," added David Sabatini, an MIT professor of biology, member of the Whitehead Institute for Biomedical Research and the Koch Institute, and also a senior author of the paper. "Interestingly, switching these cells to fatty acid oxidation enhanced their function significantly."[6]

IF may also restore microbe diversity in the gut, increase tolerance against "bad" gut microbes, and restore the integrity of the intestinal epithelium.

A study published in the *Scandinavian Journal of Immunology* found that IF (this time, alternate-day fasting for 12 weeks) helped Salmonella-infected mice clear the pathogenic bacteria more quickly through a heightened immune response.[7] Another study published in the journal *Cell Metabolism* found that every other day fasting alters the gut microbiome composition to promote an increase in the number of mitochondria in the fat tissue of mice.[8]

A study published in *Frontiers in Microbiology* in 2022 explored the impact of IF on gut microbial diversity and its associated effects on body weight and lipid profiles. The research involved 45 participants (14 women and 31 men) and analyzed blood and fecal samples collected before and after the fasting period. The study found that IF led to significant improvements in body weight and blood lipid profiles. Specifically, participants experienced an increase in high-density lipoprotein (HDL, the "good" cholesterol) and a decrease in total cholesterol, triglycerides, and low-density lipoprotein (LDL) levels. These changes were linked to favorable shifts in gut microbiota, including an increase in beneficial bacteria like *lactobacillus* and *Bifidobacterium* and a decrease in pathogenic bacteria.[9]

3. Brain Health

The (digestive) nervous system is also involved in about 30 neurotransmitters. It is estimated that 90 percent of the feel-good chemical serotonin is created in the gut. We just made the case for how fasting fixes the gut, now let's make the case for fasting for the brain.

If there's anything going on in your gut, signals are sent to your brain. This can cause unexpected symptoms and conditions, such as:

- anxiety
- depression
- stress
- schizophrenia
- other altered emotional states

If there's anything going on in the brain (like stress), it can cause symptoms in your gut, such as:

- nausea
- heartburn
- diarrhea
- constipation
- cramps
- ulcers

Brain-derived neurotrophic factor (BDNF) is like a brain fertilizer. It grows neurons and strengthens synaptic connectivity. When we are in a fasted state or high level of physical activity, we start producing more BDNF. It helps neurons grow and branch out toward each other, making it easier for them to communicate. This decreases the synaptic activity I mentioned earlier, which is very powerful. If we are *decreasing* the overall synaptic activity (the amount of communication going from neuron to neuron) but *increasing* the connectivity, we are increasing the potency of how that activity is communicated.

Imagine you have two people trying to communicate using a string-and-cup telephone, but the string is frayed and full of knots. The message gets distorted, and only a fraction of it makes it through. When you're not fasting, your neurons are like those people struggling to communicate across that tangled, fraying string. However, during fasting, your neural connections become like a clear, strong fiber-optic cable— messages travel smoothly and efficiently. With a higher percentage of energy flowing through a well-maintained, uninterrupted connection, your neurons can communicate effectively, ensuring that the signals are transmitted clearly and without loss.

BDNF not only grows neurons but also grows the connection between them. It has antidepressant activity, which explains why when you're fasting and after exercising you feel pretty damn good. The combination of BDNF and the decreased activity within the brain ends up being very powerful.

IF results in increased production of BDNF, which increases the resistance of neurons in the brain to dysfunction and degeneration in animal models of neuro-degenerative disorders. BDNF signaling may also mediate beneficial effects of IF on glucose regulation and cardiovascular function.[10]

4. Metabolism Efficiency

Many people are searching for ways to speed up their metabolism, but I doubt they want to shorten their lives in the process. Yet in the animal kingdom, the rate of living theory postulates that the faster an organism's metabolism, the shorter its lifespan. First proposed by Max Rubner in 1908, the theory was based on his observation that smaller animals had faster metabolisms and shorter lifespans compared to larger animals with slower metabolisms.

In the world of longevity, nothing extends lifespan more than caloric restriction. It's true that restricting your calories extends your lifespan, but you do this at the cost of your metabolism. Caloric restriction studies show positive outcomes for longevity in terms of reduction in blood glucose and insulin levels, sirtuin activation, and others, but it also creates a new set of problems: The metabolism and body go into starvation mode. Studies show that the immune system gets weakened, organs shrink, the thyroid slows down, and hormone imbalances occur (plus the participants in caloric restriction studies are miserable and cold all the time).[11, 12]

Won't the body go into starvation mode when you practice IF? No! A recent study shows a 13 percent increase in metabolism efficiency after four days of fasting. The human body knows what to do. When we go through a period without food, incredible processes start in the human body. There is no slowdown in metabolism. It's the complete opposite! The body starts to go into "survival mode" not "starvation mode." The body wants us to find our next meal so that we can stay alive, so it raises counter-regulatory hormones (hormones that run counter to insulin). When we don't eat food, insulin levels drop, and we raise these counter-regulatory hormones, which include catecholamines, cortisol, glucagon, and growth hormone. This is our body's way of pumping us full of energy and focus so we can hunt for our next meal.

One of the key differences between caloric restriction and intermittent fasting is their impact on metabolism. When you simply restrict calories by eating less but continue to eat throughout the day, your metabolism tends to adapt and become less efficient. In contrast, with intermittent fasting, even if you're in a calorie deficit, your metabolism doesn't slow down. Instead, it becomes more optimized due to the influence of counter-regulatory hormones.

These hormones are why our metabolism efficiency increases with fasting. Adrenaline levels are increased so that we have plenty of energy to go get more food. For example, 48 hours of fasting produces a 3.6 percent increase in metabolic rate, not the so-called "metabolic shutdown." In response to a four-day fast, resting energy expenditure increased up to 14 percent. Rather than slowing the metabolism, the body actually made it more efficient.[13]

There are three key metabolically active tissues inside your body:

1. brown adipose tissue
2. lean muscle mass
3. gut microbiome

Ancient healing strategies such as ketosis and fasting enhance all three of these important metabolically active tissues. Let's dive into all three.

Brown Adipose Tissue (BAT)

Adipose tissue is composed of fat cells, but there's a big difference between white adipose tissue (WAT) and brown adipose tissue (BAT). White fat cells store energy in the form of a single large, oily droplet. They are otherwise relatively inert. In contrast, brown fat cells contain many smaller droplets as well as mitochondria. These organelles can burn up the droplets to generate heat. Humans are mammals, and unlike reptiles we generate our own internal heat. When the body is in a cold environment, these brown fat cells become activated and literally generate heat through chemical reactions that use the oily droplets for fuel. This helps us maintain our standard operating temperature, which for most people is 98.6 degrees Fahrenheit.

Babies have BAT, presumably because they cannot yet shiver when cold, so their warmth must rely more on burning brown fat. It was long assumed that BAT disappeared in adults. However, in 2009 three different groups independently published papers in the *New England Journal of Medicine* revealing their discoveries of active brown fat cells in healthy adults. Scientists have since been trying to figure out how to study brown fat more easily and in greater detail.

Research suggests that BAT has many more benefits than WAT, mostly due to its ability to burn more energy (calories) to be used for body heat.[14, 15] During this process, your body's internal temperature increases and helps reduce other fat deposits made of WAT, the type many of us need to decrease. Certain studies have even shown that brown fat can burn up to five times more calories than other types of body fat![16]

Interestingly, because cold conditions activate brown fat, our ancestors—even those a few generations back—may have benefited from BAT's fat-burning capability because they lacked central heat. Studies have shown that people exposed to cold indoor temperatures—not super cold, just a brisk 63 degrees Fahrenheit—burn more calories from fat than people in a warmer environment.

If you want to break free from weight-loss resistance, you need to make more brown fat. The most effective way to do this is to use ketosis and fasting, along with the cutting-edge biohacks I've included later in the book—your keys to metabolic freedom.

Lean Muscle Mass

Muscle is the next metabolically active tissue inside your body that we want to prioritize. I'm not suggesting you have to become a bodybuilder, but lean muscle mass protects your metabolism in numerous ways. Muscle is mitochondrial dense, because it requires a large amount of energy to function. This is provided primarily by mitochondria in cells that consume a lot of energy.

Muscle mass helps to balance your blood sugar and insulin levels. We already discussed why high levels of blood sugar and insulin cause inflammation and weight gain—the more muscle mass you have, the more insulin sensitive you become. Think of your muscle as a sponge that mops up excess glucose out of your bloodstream, so insulin doesn't have to work as hard. This means you can enjoy yourself at the wedding or event, and your body will know what to do with the excess sugar.

When I owned my CrossFit gym back in 2015, I used to hold seminars on fasting for the members. I recall that many of them were hesitant to try fasting because they feared it would undo their hard-earned gains from working out. However, fasting actually stimulates the production of human growth hormone (HGH), which not only prevents muscle loss but also enhances your ability to build lean muscle. Far from diminishing their progress, fasting can help athletes improve their muscle development and overall fitness.

Gut Microbiome

Your gut microbiome plays a role in your metabolism, because if you're consuming 1,500 calories per day, but you only absorb 900 calories, the excess will enter your bloodstream, creating an inflammatory response. The gut microbiome plays a crucial role in regulating metabolism, influencing everything from nutrient absorption to energy balance. The diverse community of microorganisms in the gut helps break down complex carbohydrates and fibers into short-chain fatty acids (SCFAs) like butyrate, acetate, and propionate. These SCFAs not only provide energy to the cells lining the gut but also play a key role in signaling pathways that regulate fat storage, insulin sensitivity, and inflammation. By modulating these processes, the gut microbiome can directly impact metabolic health, contributing to conditions like obesity, diabetes, and cardiovascular disease when its balance is disrupted.[17, 18]

The gut microbiome interacts with various hormones and metabolites that influence hunger and satiety, such as ghrelin and leptin. A healthy gut microbiome supports the proper function of these hormones, helping to regulate appetite and prevent overeating. Dysbiosis, or an imbalance in the gut microbiome, can lead to impaired signaling and contribute to metabolic disorders like insulin resistance and metabolic syndrome. Therefore, maintaining a healthy gut microbiome is essential for optimal metabolic function and overall health.[19]

Fasting is one of the fastest ways to repair the gut microbiome. Combine this with a diet rich in SCFAs, which is included in your 30-Day Metabolic Freedom Reset, and you've got yourself the perfect recipe. This again is because fasting repairs leaky gut, allowing you to digest important vitamins and minerals for metabolic function.

You now know the extraordinary benefits that fasting has on your metabolic health, as well as its potential for treating various diseases. In the next chapter we'll look at the foods that best support your metabolism when you do break that fast.

CHAPTER 9

FOODS THAT SUPPORT YOUR METABOLISM

The right foods can ignite your metabolism, while the wrong foods can create a metabolic disaster. Food isn't the problem—it's what we've done to food that has made it problematic for our health. As we discussed in Part I, most of the food at our local supermarket has been engineered and processed, turning real food into food-like substances.

If you've been through the vicious cycle of yo-yo weight loss, it can feel like you have one foot on the gas pedal and one foot on the brakes. Eating the wrong foods at the wrong time is equivalent to putting your foot on the brakes of your metabolism. It's important to consider not the calories from the food, but the metabolic response that occurs after eating it.

In this chapter we'll examine the four key factors to consider when shopping for metabolic-boosting foods: the post-meal glucose response, the ingredients themselves, the variety of foods you eat, and the amino acid count. I'll share information about which foods to avoid as well as which ones best support your metabolism and hormones.

Key Factor 1: The Post-Meal Glucose Response

When I was obese, I noticed that I would feel extremely tired and sluggish after eating. I thought the problem was my digestive system, but the reason I felt this way was because I was eating foods that would spike my blood sugar levels. This is called "postprandial glucose" (*postprandial* means "after eating"). If there is one easy measurement you can use to help you understand the direction your health is heading, it's your blood sugar after eating. Blood sugar that is out of the healthy range can indicate metabolic disaster. As we learned in Chapter 3, high blood sugar and insulin levels lead to cardiovascular conditions like heart disease, as well as high blood pressure, elevated LDL cholesterol levels, diabetes, fatty liver disease, increasing waist circumference, and visceral fat. There are many things that influence your blood sugar, but the food you eat has the greatest impact.

You may have heard of the glycemic index, which ranks foods on a number scale of 1 to 100. Foods closer to 100 will spike your blood sugar higher than foods that rank closer to 1. This system sounds like a great way to help you navigate which foods to consume versus which foods to stay away from, but it's not as simple as it sounds. We are all unique biochemical individuals, and there are several factors that influence our blood sugar response from eating foods, such as genetics, age, health history, environment, mental health, and more.

The good news is that over the past 17 years, I've tested blood sugar levels, both fasting and postprandial, in thousands of people who have participated in my online programs or worked with me one-on-one. This extensive experience has allowed me to gather valuable insights and refine my approach to optimizing metabolic health. The data I collected, along with the research studies,[1,2] have helped me formulate the best possible foods for you to consume to balance hormones and burn fat.

We'll start with three major macronutrients: carbohydrates, proteins, and fats. Each one of these macros has a direct impact on your hormones and metabolism; they can work differently and will spike your blood sugar in unique ways.

Figure 3. Blood insulin response to different macronutrients

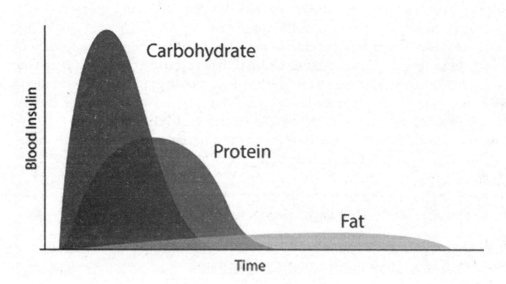

You can see in figure 3 that carbohydrates illicit the biggest blood sugar and blood insulin response after eating. Of course, whole food sources of carbohydrates will be better than processed carbohydrates, but all carbohydrates will create a glucose and insulin spike. Protein, on the other hand, has what is considered a minor, phase two insulin response. The biggest takeaway from the figure above is fat. Fat does not raise glucose and insulin at all.

The higher your postprandial glucose, the more time sugar stays in your bloodstream, creating oxidative stress and damage. Stunning as it may sound, nearly half of Americans ages 20 years and up—or more than 122 million people—have high blood pressure, according to a 2023 report from the American Heart Association.[3] Most people believe high blood pressure is a result of a diet high in salt. The belief that salt consumption raises blood pressure originates from French scientists more than 100 years ago, who "based their findings on just six patients."[4] The untold truth is that sugar is the culprit!

Having elevated blood sugar after eating inhibits the production of nitric oxide (NO). NO is a molecule produced by the body that plays a crucial role in vasodilation, helping to regulate blood flow and blood pressure. It's also involved in various cellular processes, including immune response and neurotransmission. When the blood vessels constrict because of the lack of NO from high blood sugar, the heart has to work harder. This is what increases blood pressure!

When your body has a steady supply of sugar, it will burn that and not body fat for fuel. The longer sugar remains in your bloodstream after eating, the more insulin is shuttled from your pancreas. Insulin is an energy sensor, and when it's called, the main goal is to store energy. In other words, when insulin is cranked out, your body is in a fat-storing, fed state. In simple terms, the faster you can clear sugar from your bloodstream after eating, the easier your metabolism will go into fat-burning mode.

This is why one of the first steps in your 30-Day Metabolic Freedom Reset will be to increase healthy fats and decrease carbohydrates. Healthy fats include saturated and monounsaturated fats like those found in butter, beef, eggs, seafood, avocados, and poultry. During your reset, I'll guide you on how to gradually decrease carbohydrates in a proper, sustainable way, ensuring you get the most benefit from these healthy fats. And if you currently have high blood pressure, you will notice a nice drop in your levels after just days of following your reset.

Key Factor 2: The Quality of the Ingredients

Many of us have been conditioned to look at the front label of a product, but this isn't giving us the full picture. When we walk down the grocery store aisles, we're likely to notice food products with bold, colorful labels that boast phrases like "All-Natural," "Organic," "Gluten-Free," "Low-Fat," or "High in Protein." These phrases are designed to catch our eye and make us feel like we're making a healthy choice. However, these claims often distract us from the more important information, like the actual ingredients list or nutritional facts, which may reveal hidden sugars, unhealthy fats, or artificial additives. This conditioning leads us to focus on the appealing front-of-label marketing rather than the detailed facts that could affect our health.

It's very important to read the full ingredients list on the back of the label. Real food will have only a few ingredients. If you think about it, when you buy an avocado or eggs, there's no list of ingredients on the label. It's what you see in front of you: the avocado or the egg.

When a whole food is processed, it becomes insulinogenic. Insulinogenic refers to the capacity of a food or substance to stimulate insulin production in the body. Take an apple, for instance. In its whole form, it's rich in fiber, vitamins, and natural sugars. When processed into juice, however, much of the fiber is removed, leaving mainly the sugars and some vitamins. In their whole form, potatoes provide fiber, vitamins, and minerals. Yet when processed into chips, they are often fried in unhealthy oils and coated with salt, significantly increasing the calorie and sodium content while reducing nutritional benefits.

When you eat foods that have a list of healthy ingredients, such as the right fats and proteins, they support hormonal production, while fake "frankenfoods" have chemical-laden ingredients that have been associated with disrupting your hormones, which leads to a metabolic nightmare. Keep in mind that every bite of food is either feeding disease or supporting wellness. If you see a long list of ingredients with items you can't pronounce, these are red flags of synthetic junk that will disrupt your metabolic health.

Ingredients Toxic to Your Metabolism

The sad truth is that many "healthy" foods are not safe for your metabolism. Companies are focusing on profits and shelf life over health and wellness. There has been a rapid rise in toxic ingredients in food, and if your priority is a healthy metabolism, it's pertinent to be aware of them. Preservatives, artificial sweeteners, pesticides, dyes, and artificial flavors are all common ingredients on food labels. As for the terms "fat free" and "all natural," they might as well be associated with the term "chemical shitstorm."

It can be difficult to wrap your head around the fact that toxic ingredients can disrupt your metabolism, but once you're aware, you can make better decisions. Italy and many other countries in Europe have banned several of these toxic ingredients, such as red dyes and pesticides, but here in the United States our regulations are loose. In fact, many processed foods sold in the United States have different ingredients in Europe because of their strict regulations. For example, cereals in the United States often include artificial dyes like Yellow #5 and Red #40, while European versions use natural colorings such as turmeric. In the United States, soft drinks like Mountain Dew contain brominated vegetable oil (BVO), which is banned in Europe over health concerns. Even fast food items differ—McDonald's fries in the United States have preservatives and anti-foaming agents like dimethylpolysiloxane that are omitted in European versions.

In the United States, "Generally Recognized as Safe" (GRAS) is a designation for substances added to food that are considered safe by experts, based on a long history of common use in food or on the results of scientific research. The GRAS designation is a key part of the regulatory framework overseen by the Food and Drug Administration (FDA). Substances that are GRAS do not require pre-market approval by the FDA, although they must meet the same safety standards as approved food additives.

GRAS status can be self-determined by manufacturers, but they must provide evidence of safety, and the FDA can review and challenge these determinations. This system aims to ensure the safety of the food supply while allowing for innovation and the introduction of new food ingredients. Because of this, if there is no clear evidence of harm, despite the lack of long-term research, the ingredient can be categorized as GRAS.

Let's take a look at some of the ingredients most toxic to your metabolism.

The Potential Health Hazards of Apeel

Apeel, a plant-based coating applied to fresh produce to extend shelf life, has raised several health concerns among consumers. Here are some key points:

- **Chemical composition:** Apeel consists mainly of purified monoglycerides and diglycerides derived from vegetable oils. While these substances occur naturally and are used in other food applications, their production involves chemical processes that raise concerns about potential contaminants, including trace amounts of heavy metals like palladium, arsenic, lead, cadmium, and mercury. Although these levels are within safety standards set by the United States and European Union, the cumulative effects of long-term exposure remain unclear.

- **Regulatory and transparency issues:** Apeel is classified as a food additive, which means it undergoes a different approval process than pesticides. This classification allows for a degree of self-regulation, where companies can determine the safety of their products without extensive external oversight. This has led to concerns about the adequacy of safety testing and the transparency of the ingredients used in the coating.

- **Potential health risks:** There are claims that edible coatings like Apeel could pose risks to individuals with allergies, sensitivities, and certain chronic illnesses. The lack of labeling requirements for these coatings means consumers may be unaware of what they are ingesting, which is particularly concerning for those who rely on organic foods to avoid additives and allergens.[5]

- **Nutrient impact:** While Apeel helps maintain the moisture and appearance of produce, there are questions about its impact on the nutrient density of the coated fruits and vegetables. The coatings might alter the natural microbiome of the produce, potentially affecting its overall nutritional value.

To avoid purchasing fruits and vegetables coated with Apeel, it's important to be vigilant about where and how you shop. Start by carefully checking labels and stickers on produce for any mention of "Apeel" or similar terms like "Edipeel," as these indicate the presence of the protective coating. Shopping at farmers' markets or directly from local growers is another effective strategy, as these sources often offer produce that hasn't been treated with commercial coatings. Additionally, many organic suppliers avoid using such treatments, so opting for organic produce might help you steer clear of Apeel, though it's still wise to confirm with the supplier. When in doubt, don't hesitate to ask store employees or produce managers for more information about the products they sell. By taking these steps, you can better ensure that the fruits and vegetables you purchase align with your preferences for natural, untreated produce.

The Health Dangers of Processed Meats

A study published in 1994 found that children who consume more than 12 hot dogs per month have a significantly increased risk of developing childhood leukemia, with the risk being nine times higher compared to children who consume fewer hot dogs. This study suggests a potential link between the consumption of processed meats, which contain nitrites, and the development of leukemia. The results indicate that high intake of such processed meats could be a contributing factor to childhood leukemia, although more research is needed to confirm these findings.[6]

And, to make it worse, certain processed meats such as hot dogs can also contain other harmful chemicals that can form when meat is cooked at high temperatures. These toxic ingredients include nitrites and nitrates, artificial flavors and colors, phosphates, and trans fats. One study found that just half a hot dog a day upped breast cancer risk by 21 percent.[7] The consumption of processed meats, such as hot dogs, poses significant risks not only to cancer development but also to metabolic health. The presence of harmful chemicals like nitrites, nitrates, and trans fats in these foods can contribute to metabolic dysfunction, leading to insulin resistance, inflammation, and oxidative stress. These factors disrupt normal metabolic processes and may increase the risk of obesity, type 2 diabetes, and other metabolic disorders.

High-Fructose Corn Syrup

There's another hidden ingredient in most foods that puts the brakes on fat loss because of its dangerous effect on mitochondria. It's found in many "healthy" products and can even be called different names. You've already learned that mitochondria are the powerhouses of the cell, but let's delve into how they help you burn belly fat.

Mitochondria are responsible for producing an energy currency called adenosine triphosphate (ATP). When your mitochondria are healthy, they generate a substantial amount of ATP, which not only energizes you but also increases heat production in your body. This heightened energy demand and heat production elevate your basal metabolic rate (BMR), which means you burn more calories at rest, without the need for additional exercise or calorie counting. Essentially, healthy mitochondria enable you to burn more belly fat while simply sitting on the couch! However, there's a common ingredient in many diets that acts as a mitochondrial poison: high-fructose corn syrup (HFCS).

HFCS is a common sweetener that has profound effects on our metabolic health. When HFCS impairs mitochondrial function, it reduces ATP production, leading to a slower, inefficient metabolism. This impairment also increases cellular inflammation, which interferes with the body's ability to burn fat effectively.[8, 9] Another significant concern with HFCS is its failure to trigger satiety, the feeling of fullness that tells us to stop eating.[10] Unlike other nutrients that signal our brain to reduce food intake, HFCS bypasses this mechanism, leading to overeating and subsequent weight gain. This lack of satiety is particularly problematic as it encourages excessive calorie consumption, making it difficult to maintain a healthy weight.

HFCS also plays a detrimental role in insulin resistance.[11, 12] High intake of this sweetener makes the body's cells less responsive to insulin, resulting in elevated blood sugar levels. Over time, this condition can lead to increased fat storage, especially around the abdomen, which is a risk factor for various metabolic disorders. The body's inability to process insulin efficiently creates a cascade of metabolic issues that contribute to obesity and other health problems.

Moreover, fructose, a major component of HFCS, is primarily metabolized in the liver.[13] When consumed in large quantities, fructose is converted into fat, leading to liver fat accumulation and overall body fat increase. This process not only contributes to weight gain but also poses significant risks to liver health, further complicating metabolic functions.

HFCS disrupts the balance of hunger hormones like leptin and ghrelin. These hormones play crucial roles in regulating appetite and energy balance. When their normal functioning is disturbed, it can lead to increased appetite and cravings, making it difficult to stop eating. This hormonal imbalance is a significant barrier to weight loss and overall metabolic health.

The consumption of HFCS is also linked to metabolic syndrome, a cluster of conditions including increased blood pressure, high blood sugar, excess body fat around the waist, and abnormal cholesterol levels.[14, 15] This syndrome significantly increases the risk of cardiovascular disease, diabetes, and other serious health issues. The metabolic disruptions caused by HFCS make it extremely challenging to manage weight effectively and maintain good health.

Additionally, HFCS can elevate triglyceride levels in the blood.[16] High triglyceride levels are associated with an increased risk of heart disease and contribute to fat storage, particularly in the abdominal area. This promotes weight gain and further complicates efforts to achieve a healthy body weight.

Lastly, HFCS intake can lead to oxidative stress and inflammation in the body.[17] Chronic inflammation is a known factor in the development of obesity and other metabolic disorders. By interfering with metabolic processes, oxidative stress and inflammation make it harder for the body to lose weight and maintain a healthy metabolism.

Understanding the impact of HFCS on your metabolism and overall health is crucial. Avoiding this ingredient can help maintain healthy mitochondrial function, improve your metabolism, and support your weight-loss goals. Some of the ingredients with different names that contain HFCS include:

- corn syrup
- glucose-fructose syrup
- isoglucose
- maize syrup
- tapioca syrup
- fruit fructose
- glucose syrup
- high-fructose maize syrup

Here are the top 10 most common "health" foods that contain high-fructose corn syrup:

1. flavored yogurts
2. granola bars
3. protein bars
4. breakfast cereals
5. smoothies
6. fruit juices
7. salad dressings
8. whole wheat and multigrain breads
9. sports drinks
10. instant oatmeal

QUESTIONS TO CONSIDER WHEN SHOPPING

There's a ton of moving parts when shopping for healthy food, and it can be overwhelming and confusing. You can ask yourself the following questions to help you avoid purchasing foods that disrupt your metabolism:

- How long is the ingredients list?
- Are there any ingredients that you cannot pronounce?
- Do they contain the bad oils mentioned in this book?
- Do you see any artificial colors, flavors, or dyes listed?
- Does it contain HFCS?

Metabolism-Supporting Foods

Once you become aware of the toxic ingredients to avoid, you can focus on adding in the foods that boost your metabolism. When you eat real foods that support your metabolic health, the body naturally lowers inflammation, balances hormones, and burns stubborn fat. The highest-quality foods don't require an ingredients list because what you see is what you get. For example, beef, avocados, and berries don't have an ingredients list because they're in their original form. You'll find most of these whole foods in the perimeter of the grocery store instead of the inner aisles. This is where you'll be able to avoid chemical-laden frankenfoods to give your body the best chance at health.

Real, high-quality foods fall into three categories:

1. They support your metabolism.

2. They rebuild your gut microbiome.

3. They build your lean muscle.

Hormones play an important role in your metabolism. They are simply chemical messengers communicating with every cell inside your body. For example, your sex hormones—estrogen and testosterone—are hugely influenced by what you eat (and don't eat). It's not just your sex hormones—the hormone adiponectin, released by fat cells, plays a role in fat loss by aiding in the breakdown of body fat. Understanding what builds each of these hormones will give your body a metabolic advantage.

Estrogen

You build estrogen when you lower glucose and insulin levels. This means ordering the burger without the bun—the starchy carbohydrates from the bun spike blood sugar and cause estrogen to go into hiding.

Low estrogen levels can significantly impact a woman's health and well-being, such as through these five common symptoms:

1. hot flashes, which are sudden feelings of warmth often accompanied by sweating and reddening of the skin

2. night sweats, a similar phenomenon that occurs during sleep and can disrupt rest and contribute to fatigue

3. vaginal dryness, which can lead to discomfort and pain during intercourse

4. mood swings, including feelings of irritability, depression, and anxiety

5. decreased bone density, which can increase the risk of osteoporosis and fractures

While the symptoms might differ from those in women, low estrogen levels in men can also have significant health implications. One common symptom is reduced libido, leading to a decrease in sexual desire and activity. Men may also experience erectile dysfunction, making it difficult to achieve or maintain an erection. Another symptom is fatigue, characterized by a persistent feeling of tiredness and lack of energy. Mood changes, such as increased irritability, depression, and anxiety, are also common. Additionally, low estrogen levels can contribute to decreased bone density, increasing the risk of fractures and osteoporosis.

While low estrogen isn't good, neither is too much—it's all about maintaining the right balance. Estrogen dominance has skyrocketed over the years thanks to endocrine-disrupting chemicals (EDCs) that can interfere with the body's endocrine system, which regulates hormones. These substances can mimic, block, or alter the normal function of hormones, leading to a range of health issues. Endocrine disruptors can be found in various sources, including pesticides, plastics, cosmetics, and even some food and water supplies.

This is one of many reasons why I love the ketogenic lifestyle paired with intermittent fasting. Ketosis and fasting work powerfully together to balance estrogen because of their impact on reducing glucose and insulin levels inside the body. Outside of a low-carbohydrate, keto approach, there are several foods that can help balance your estrogen levels. Healthy fats would be right at the top of my list because they contain healthy cholesterol, which is the precursor to building estrogen. If the thought of eating cholesterol scares you, you aren't alone. Many people are dealing with lipophobia—the fear of dietary fat, based on 50-plus years of propaganda and misinformation.

The hypothesis that cholesterol causes heart disease started in the 1950s when researchers began to explore the connection between dietary fat, cholesterol, and heart disease. Ancel Keys, an American physiologist, played a pivotal role in promoting this hypothesis. His influential "Seven Countries Study" (the United States, Finland, Italy, Greece, Yugoslavia [now primarily Serbia and Croatia], the Netherlands, and Japan), which began in the late 1950s and was published in the 1970s, suggested a correlation between dietary saturated fat intake, serum cholesterol levels, and the incidence of heart disease. What Ancel Keys didn't publish was the 15 other countries that did not fit his theory. In addition to the Seven Countries Study, Ancel Keys initially gathered data from 15 other countries in his broader 22-country analysis: Australia, Canada, Chile, England, Germany, Guatemala, India, Ireland, Israel, Mexico, the Philippines, Portugal, South Africa, Sweden, and Switzerland. These countries did not align with his hypothesis, so he excluded this data from his final analysis.[18]

Before Ancel Keys's research gained attention, autopsies of heart attack victims had already consistently shown substantial atherosclerotic plaques—buildups of cholesterol and fatty deposits—in their coronary arteries. In 1912, Dr. James Herrick conducted a landmark study that first identified the link between coronary thrombosis and myocardial infarction.[19] During autopsies of heart attack victims, researchers and pathologists observed that many of these individuals had significant amounts of cholesterol and fatty deposits, known as atherosclerotic plaques, in their arteries. These plaques were found to narrow the arteries, reducing blood flow and increasing the risk of blockages. The plaques were primarily composed of cholesterol, fatty substances, cellular waste products, calcium, and fibrin (a clotting material in the blood); therefore, the researchers concluded that cholesterol was the cause of the narrowing of the arteries, leading to heart disease.

Just as it would be misguided to conclude that firefighters cause fires simply because they are consistently found at fire scenes, it might be equally misguided to blame cholesterol solely for causing heart attacks merely because it is present in atherosclerotic plaques. In both cases, the presence can be seen as responses to a problem rather than the root cause. Firefighters are there to extinguish fires and mitigate damage, not start fires. Similarly, cholesterol might accumulate in arteries as part of the body's response to underlying issues like inflammation, arterial damage, or other factors that contribute to heart disease. When you eat the right fats, it raises your HDL cholesterol, which is protective and lowers inflammation inside your body.

In addition to healthy fats, estrogen loves healthy phytoestrogens, which are naturally occurring compounds found in certain plants. Phytoestrogens can mimic or modulate the body's estrogen levels, helping to maintain hormonal balance. Consuming foods rich in them, such as soy products, flaxseeds, sesame seeds, and legumes, can help alleviate symptoms of hormonal imbalances like hot flashes, mood swings, and irregular menstrual cycles.

FOODS THAT SUPPORT ESTROGEN

Good Fats

- salmon
- sardines
- mackerel
- avocados
- avocado oil
- olives
- olive oil
- sesame seed oil

- flaxseed oil
- coriander oil
- coconut and coconut oil

- MCT oil
- grass-fed butter
- grass-fed ghee

Fruits and Vegetables

- pomegranates
- blueberries
- strawberries
- cranberries
- apples
- plums
- peaches
- broccoli

- cauliflower
- Brussels sprouts
- carrots
- sweet potatoes
- cabbage
- sprouts
- onion
- garlic

Seeds and Nuts

- flaxseeds
- sesame seeds
- sunflower seeds
- pumpkin seeds
- chia seeds

- walnuts
- pistachios
- Brazil nuts
- cashews
- pine nuts

Legumes

- chickpeas
- lentils
- black beans
- kidney beans

- peas
- pinto beans
- mung beans
- black-eyed peas

Testosterone

Testosterone is another hormone that is highly influenced by food choices. While males have more testosterone than females—and most people think of it as a male sex hormone—female adrenal glands and ovaries produce small amounts. Women lose testosterone during menopause, and because testosterone helps build muscle and burn calories, this hormone imbalance leads to muscle loss, lower metabolism, and weight gain.

Adequate levels of testosterone support muscle mass maintenance and growth, which in turn boosts the metabolic rate and promotes fat burning. This hormone also enhances energy levels, motivation, and physical performance, making regular exercise more effective for weight management. Additionally, testosterone helps regulate the distribution of body fat, reducing the accumulation of visceral fat, which is associated with various health risks. Beyond its role in fat loss, testosterone contributes to bone density, cardiovascular health, and overall mood and cognitive function. Maintaining healthy levels is essential for achieving and sustaining optimal health and well-being.

In men, testosterone levels typically peak during adolescence and early adulthood. After the age of 30, testosterone begins to decline at an average rate of about 1 percent per year. By the time men reach their 70s and 80s, their testosterone levels can be significantly lower than during their younger years. This gradual decline can lead to symptoms such as decreased muscle mass, increased body fat, reduced libido, and lower energy levels.[20, 21]

In women, testosterone levels also peak in early adulthood and start to decline as they age. However, the decline is usually more gradual and less pronounced than in men. Testosterone in women drops by about 50 percent between the ages of 20 and 40. After menopause, women experience a further decline. By the time women reach their 70s and 80s, their testosterone levels can be very low, contributing to reduced muscle mass, decreased bone density, and changes in mood and energy levels.[22]

You can naturally boost your testosterone levels by adding in the following foods.

FOODS THAT SUPPORT TESTOSTERONE

Fats and Protiens

- eggs
- avocados
- salmon
- anchovies
- sardines
- mackerel
- red meat
- olive oil

Fruits and Vegetables

- pomegranates
- arugula
- Swiss chard
- garlic
- onions

Seeds and Nuts

- Brazil nuts
- pumpkin seeds
- walnuts
- macadamia nuts

Adiponectin

Adiponectin is a hormone produced by adipose (fat) tissue that plays a crucial role in regulating glucose levels and fatty acid breakdown. It enhances insulin sensitivity, making it easier for cells to absorb glucose from the bloodstream, thus helping to maintain healthy blood sugar levels. In terms of fat loss, adiponectin boosts the body's ability to break down fat and reduces the accumulation of fat cells. It supports skin health as well: Adiponectin has anti-inflammatory properties that help protect the skin from damage caused by inflammation and oxidative stress; it also supports collagen production, essential for maintaining skin elasticity and reducing the appearance of wrinkles. By promoting better metabolism and reducing inflammation, adiponectin contributes to overall skin vitality and a healthier body composition.

Think of adiponectin as a diligent traffic cop in a neighborhood intersection. Just as a traffic cop ensures smooth and efficient movement of vehicles through intersections, adiponectin regulates the flow and usage of energy in the body. When traffic is light and moving smoothly, the traffic cop may relax but always remains vigilant, ready to step in when necessary. In times of heavy traffic, like during rush hour, the traffic cop actively directs vehicles to prevent jams and accidents. In the body, during periods of increased energy demand or stress, adiponectin enhances insulin sensitivity and stimulates the breakdown of fatty acids, preventing the buildup of fat and maintaining smooth metabolic function. This regulation helps prevent metabolic "traffic jams" that can lead to conditions like insulin resistance and type 2 diabetes.

By efficiently managing the "traffic" of glucose and fats, adiponectin ensures that energy flow remains steady and cells function optimally, contributing to overall metabolic health. You can activate it through exercise or by consuming any of these foods:

1. olive oil
2. wild-caught fish
3. olives
4. avocados
5. berries

Foods That Rebuild Your Gut Microbiome

Believe it or not, we have 10 times more bacterial cells than human cells, and most bacteria in the gut have 100 to 150 more genes than the human genome. This makes me ponder the question, are we humans with bacteria or are we bacteria having a human experience?

When you eat the right foods, you power up the good bacteria inside your gut microbiome, which helps your metabolism function, balances hormones for fat loss, and allows your brain to make neurotransmitters. Ninety percent of all the bacteria that live in your body exists in your gut. In fact, the majority of your immune system is inside your digestive tract. So when you consume inflammatory foods such as seed oils, sugars, and chemical-laden ingredients, you kill your good bacteria and create an environment for bad bacteria to flourish. The great news is that you can bring healthy bacteria back in only a matter of days.

Bacteria thrive when these four conditions are met: a hormetic stress via fasting and consuming probiotic, prebiotic, and polyphenol foods. It may surprise you to learn that a positive stress like fasting helps create diversity in your gut microbiome.

As you recall, not all stress is bad. When you are in a fasted state, adaptation is the name of the game. The stress of not having food energy available through digestion creates a hormetic stress that signals an adaptation response toward your bacteria. This increases microbial diversity in which good bacteria flourish and bad bacteria don't survive. It's survival of the fittest right inside your gut microbiome!

ANTIBIOTICS AND OTHER GUT DISRUPTORS

Antibiotics, while sometimes essential for fighting bacterial infections, can significantly disrupt gut diversity by indiscriminately killing both harmful *and* beneficial bacteria. Taking antibiotics is akin to dropping a bomb on an entire city to kill one bad guy: In the same way that a bomb indiscriminately destroys everything in its path, obliterating both the enemy and innocent civilians alike, antibiotics annihilate both harmful pathogens and beneficial bacteria in the gut. This widespread destruction leaves the microbial environment devastated, wiping out the good bacteria that are essential for maintaining a healthy, balanced microbiome. Just as a city needs time to rebuild after such a catastrophic event, the gut requires time and care to restore its microbial diversity and regain its functional harmony after a course of antibiotics. This reduction in diversity weakens the gut microbiome, compromising its ability to support digestion, immune function, and overall health.

Other factors contributing to the loss of gut diversity include a poor diet high in processed foods and low in fiber, chronic stress, the birth control pill, lack of physical activity, and environmental toxins. These elements can further harm the delicate balance of bacteria, leading to issues such as digestive disorders, weakened immune response, and increased susceptibility to chronic diseases. Adding in probiotic-rich foods is the quickest way to restore the beautiful city inside your gut microbiome.

Probiotic-Rich Foods

Probiotic foods play a crucial role in maintaining a healthy gut microbiome, which is essential for overall health and well-being. These foods, rich in beneficial bacteria, help balance the gut flora by enhancing the population of good microbes. Regular consumption of probiotic-rich foods—such as yogurt, kefir, sauerkraut, kimchi, and other fermented products—can reduce inflammation, support metabolic health, and even influence mental health by producing neurotransmitters like serotonin. By fostering a diverse and robust microbial community, probiotic foods help prevent gastrointestinal issues, support healthy weight management, and protect against various chronic diseases. Incorporating these foods into your diet is a natural and effective way to nurture your gut health and promote overall vitality.

The fermentation process is a natural method of food preservation that involves the breakdown of sugars by bacteria, yeasts, or other microorganisms. During fermentation, these microorganisms consume sugars and convert them into alcohol, gases, or organic acids. This not only extends the shelf life of the food but also enhances its nutritional profile and creates probiotic-rich products. The beneficial bacteria produced during fermentation, such as the lactobacillus and Bifidobacterium species, play a crucial role in maintaining a healthy gut microbiome—they help to outcompete harmful bacteria, reduce inflammation, and promote digestive health by maintaining the integrity of the gut lining.

Fermentation also helps break down sugars in foods, resulting in a lower glycemic load. As the microorganisms consume the sugars, they reduce the overall carbohydrate content of the food, leading to a slower and more gradual release of glucose into the bloodstream. This process helps in stabilizing blood sugar levels and can be particularly beneficial for individuals with insulin resistance or diabetes. By lowering the glycemic load, fermented foods can prevent spikes in blood sugar and insulin levels, which are often linked to weight gain and metabolic disorders. Incorporating fermented foods into your diet not only supports gut health but also contributes to better blood sugar management, making it a valuable strategy for maintaining overall metabolic health.

Each food you ferment can provide different healing benefits. For example, sauerkraut, a fermented cabbage dish, offers numerous health benefits due to its rich probiotic content and high nutrient density. The fermentation process enhances the availability of beneficial bacteria, which support a healthy gut microbiome, improve digestion, and boost immune function. Additionally, sauerkraut is packed with vitamins C and K, fiber, and various antioxidants that contribute to overall health. Regular consumption of sauerkraut can help reduce inflammation, promote heart health, and even support mental well-being by fostering a balanced gut-brain connection. Including sauerkraut in your diet is a delicious and natural way to enhance your nutritional intake and support overall vitality.

Thankfully, fermented foods have become popular, and you can find all kinds of them at your local grocery store.

PROBIOTIC-RICH FERMENTED FOODS

- yogurt
- sauerkraut
- pickles
- kimchi
- kombucha

- kefir dairy
- kefir water
- natto
- tempeh

Prebiotic-Rich Foods

Prebiotic-rich foods are essential for maintaining a healthy gut microbiome, because they provide the necessary nutrients to feed beneficial bacteria. Prebiotic foods are like the fertilizer for a garden, nourishing the soil so that healthy plants (probiotics) can grow and thrive. Just as fertilizer provides essential nutrients that help plants flourish, prebiotic foods supply the vital fibers that beneficial gut bacteria need to multiply and support a robust and balanced gut microbiome. This enriched environment allows the "good" bacteria to outcompete harmful invaders, promoting overall digestive health and well-being. These foods, which include garlic, onions, leeks, asparagus, bananas, and whole grains, contain nondigestible fibers that promote the growth and activity of probiotics in the gut.

By enhancing the proliferation of good bacteria, prebiotics help improve digestion, boost immune function, and enhance nutrient absorption. A diet rich in them can help reduce inflammation, regulate bowel movements, and support overall metabolic health.

PREBIOTIC FOODS

- garlic
- onions
- leeks
- asparagus

- bananas
- chicory root
- Jerusalem artichokes
- dandelion greens

- pistachios
- split peas
- red kidney beans
- cashews
- oats
- apples

- konjac root
- burdock root
- seaweed
- flaxseeds
- cocoa

Polyphenol Foods

Polyphenol-rich foods offer significant benefits for the gut microbiome by fostering a diverse and healthy population of beneficial bacteria. These compounds, found abundantly in fruits, vegetables, tea, coffee, red wine, and dark chocolate, act as prebiotics, providing nourishment for beneficial gut microbes. When consumed, polyphenols undergo partial digestion in the small intestine, with the remaining compounds reaching the colon, where they are metabolized by gut bacteria. This process not only promotes the growth of good bacteria but also helps suppress the proliferation of harmful bacteria, leading to a balanced and resilient gut microbiome.

Polyphenols possess strong anti-inflammatory and antioxidant properties that contribute to gut health. Chronic inflammation and oxidative stress in the gut can disrupt the microbial balance and damage the intestinal lining, leading to various gastrointestinal disorders. By reducing inflammation and neutralizing harmful free radicals, polyphenols help protect the gut environment, supporting the integrity of the intestinal barrier and promoting overall digestive health.

Additionally, polyphenol-rich foods can enhance the production of beneficial short-chain fatty acids (SCFAs), such as butyrate, propionate, and acetate. These SCFAs are produced by gut bacteria during the fermentation of polyphenols and other fibers, and they play a crucial role in maintaining gut health. SCFAs provide energy for colon cells, reduce inflammation, and support the immune system. The presence of SCFAs in the gut is associated with a lower risk of gastrointestinal diseases, improved metabolic health, and a stronger immune response, highlighting the importance of polyphenol-rich foods in a balanced diet.

Polyphenol-rich foods support a healthy gut microbiome by nourishing beneficial bacteria, which then produce short-chain fatty acids (SCFAs). These SCFAs strengthen the intestinal lining, reduce inflammation, and maintain a balanced gut environment, helping to suppress harmful bacteria and protect against gastrointestinal disorders. In essence, polyphenols help your gut microbiome stay balanced, resilient, and functioning at its best.

POLYPHENOL FOODS

- blueberries
- dark chocolate
- blackberries
- strawberries
- raspberries
- green tea
- black tea
- artichoke hearts
- broccoli
- red onions
- olives
- extra virgin olive oil
- walnuts
- pecans

- coffee
- turmeric
- cranberries
- shallots
- Brussels sprouts
- saffron
- oregano
- thyme
- basil
- parsley
- cinnamon
- cumin
- curry

As you incorporate these microbiome-rebuilding foods, you'll notice your taste buds begin to shift. For most of my life, my gut microbiome and brain craved sugar and processed carbohydrates, because I had trained them by eating these unhealthy foods on a daily basis. The obese version of myself would have never thought that I'd be able to overcome those cravings and switch my palate to crave microbiome-building foods instead. However, the shift did happen for me, and it happened within days. If I was able to rearrange my taste buds, you can do it too. When you are consistent with eating the foods I've outlined here, you will support hormone production, turn on fat burning, and power up your gut microbiome.

Key Factor 3: The Variety of the Foods You Eat

When it comes to metabolic health, gut diversity is king, queen, and everything in between. I've surveyed hundreds of students in the past. I'd ask them to journal how many different foods they have on a weekly basis. To my surprise, most of them ate the same eight foods over and over. Limiting food choices can restrict the growth of helpful microbes. Our microbes work with our hormones and metabolism to create a thriving environment, and if we don't give them the building blocks they need to thrive, then symptoms will manifest as the body's way of communicating with us.

Different foods contain various nutrients that feed distinct bacteria in the gut, promoting a diverse and balanced microbiome. For instance, fiber-rich foods like beans, lentils, and whole grains provide soluble fiber that nourishes beneficial bacteria like Bifidobacteria and lactobacilli. These bacteria ferment the fiber, producing short-chain fatty acids (SCFAs) such as butyrate, which support gut health and reduce inflammation. Prebiotic foods like garlic, onions, and leeks contain inulin and fructooligosaccharides (FOS), which specifically feed these beneficial bacteria, enhancing their growth and activity. Polyphenol-rich foods like berries, dark chocolate, and green tea offer antioxidants that also serve as prebiotics, fostering the growth of good bacteria while suppressing harmful strains. This nutrient diversity is crucial for maintaining a robust and healthy gut microbiome.

Diet variation, as emphasized by my mentor Dr. Daniel Pompa, author of *The Cellular Healing Diet*, is the practice of regularly changing the types and amounts of foods you eat to optimize health and metabolic function. This approach aligns with ancestral eating patterns, where humans had to adapt to seasonal changes and varying food availability. By mimicking these natural cycles, diet variation can help break metabolic plateaus, enhance metabolic flexibility, and promote overall health.

One of the core principles of diet variation is seasonal eating. Consuming foods that are in season ensures that you are obtaining the freshest and most nutrient-dense produce. In the summer, for example, focus on light, hydrating fruits and vegetables, while in the winter, incorporate more hearty, warming foods. Seasonal eating not only provides a diverse array of nutrients but also helps your body adapt to environmental changes, enhancing immune function and overall resilience.

Diet variation includes periodic fasting and feasting cycles. By alternating periods of low-calorie intake with times of higher calorie consumption, you can boost your metabolism and improve cellular health. This cyclical approach can help reset hormonal balances, reduce inflammation, and support the body's natural detoxification processes. Embracing diet variation encourages a dynamic approach to eating that can lead to sustainable health improvements and greater vitality.

Incorporating a variety of fresh or dried spices into your diet is an excellent way to increase food diversity and reap numerous health benefits. Spices such as turmeric, cumin, ginger, and cinnamon are rich in antioxidants, anti-inflammatory compounds, and essential nutrients. These spices not only enhance the flavor of your meals but also support gut health by promoting the growth of beneficial bacteria and suppressing harmful ones. Regularly consuming a diverse array of spices can improve digestion, boost metabolism, and strengthen the immune system, contributing to overall well-being and vitality. Add the following spices to your diet:

- turmeric
- cumin
- ginger
- cinnamon
- black pepper
- garlic
- onion powder
- paprika
- cayenne pepper
- cardamom
- cloves
- coriander
- fennel seeds
- mustard seeds
- nutmeg
- oregano
- rosemary
- sage
- thyme
- basil

Key Factor 4: Amino Acid Count

Amino acid count is simply a fancy way of saying high-quality protein. Amino acids are crucial for building healthy bodies. Dr. Gabrielle Lyon's book *Forever Strong: A New, Science-Based Strategy for Aging Well* highlights a crucial yet often overlooked aspect of the obesity epidemic: the issue of being *undermuscled*. According to Dr. Lyon, the root cause of many metabolic problems, including obesity, is not merely excess fat but a deficiency in muscle mass. She argues that we are facing a "muscle crisis," where the lack of sufficient muscle tissue contributes significantly to poor metabolic health and the rising rates of obesity.

Muscle tissue is metabolically active and plays a key role in energy expenditure. It burns calories even at rest, meaning that higher muscle mass can significantly boost basal metabolic rate. When people are undermuscled, their bodies become less efficient at burning calories, leading to easier fat accumulation and weight gain. Dr. Lyon emphasizes that muscle is the key to longevity and that building muscle is critical for improving metabolic health and combating obesity. Moreover, Dr. Lyon's research points out that muscle acts as a regulator of glucose metabolism. Adequate muscle mass helps in the effective disposal of glucose, thereby preventing insulin resistance, a common precursor to obesity and type 2 diabetes.

By prioritizing muscle health through resistance training and protein-rich diets, individuals can enhance their metabolic health, increase their energy expenditure, and more effectively manage their weight. Dr. Lyon's approach suggests that building and maintaining muscle mass is a powerful strategy in addressing the obesity epidemic and improving overall health.

Additionally, the protein leverage hypothesis states that human beings will prioritize the consumption of protein in food over other dietary components and will eat until protein needs have been met, regardless of energy content,[23] thus leading to overconsumption of foodstuffs when their protein content is low. This hypothesis has been put forward as a potential explanation for the obesity epidemic. Empirical tests have provided some evidence to confirm the hypothesis, with one study suggesting that this could be a link between ultra-processed foods and the prevalence of obesity in the developed world.

In 1995, Australian researcher Susanna Holt developed the concept of *satiety value*, a measure of how much a given food is likely to satisfy someone's hunger. High-protein foods have been found to have high satiety values.[24]

There are three specific amino acids we want to eat: leucine, isoleucine, and valine. These essential branched-chain amino acids (BCAAs) play a vital role in muscle protein synthesis, energy production, and overall muscle health. They cannot be synthesized by the body and must be obtained through diet. Rich sources of BCAAs include high-protein foods, such as meat, poultry, fish, eggs, dairy products, and plant-based options like legumes, soy products, nuts, and seeds. Incorporating these foods into your diet ensures an adequate intake of leucine, isoleucine, and valine, supporting muscle growth, cellular repair, and overall metabolic health.

As I mentioned earlier, muscle acts like a sponge for glucose, soaking up sugar from the bloodstream and storing it for energy. Just as a sponge absorbs water efficiently, muscle tissue takes in glucose, preventing excess sugar from accumulating in the blood. This absorption helps regulate blood sugar levels and keeps your metabolism running smoothly. When you have more lean muscle, your body can manage glucose better, reducing the risk of insulin resistance and related health issues, much like a larger sponge can absorb more water, keeping surfaces clean and dry.

LEAN MUSCLE AMINO ACID FOODS

- chicken
- beef
- fish
- pork
- eggs
- Greek yogurt
- cottage cheese
- tofu
- lentils
- pumpkin seeds
- quinoa
- edamame

When consuming both animal and plant-based foods, it's important to make sure these foods are organic, non-GMO, and antibiotic free. This is crucial for maximizing health benefits and minimizing exposure to harmful substances. Organic foods are grown without synthetic pesticides and fertilizers, reducing the risk of ingesting potentially toxic chemicals. Non-GMO foods ensure that you are not consuming genetically modified organisms, which may have unknown long-term health effects. Antibiotic-free animal products help prevent the ingestion of antibiotic residues, which can contribute to antibiotic resistance and disrupt gut microbiota. Choosing organic, non-GMO, and antibiotic-free options supports a cleaner diet and promotes a healthier metabolism.

Eating the right amount of amino acids triggers a process in your body called mTOR, or the mechanistic target of rapamycin. This is a crucial cellular pathway that regulates growth, metabolism, and protein synthesis in the body. It acts as a central hub, integrating signals from nutrients, growth factors, and energy status to control cell growth and proliferation.

Imagine mTOR as a building supervisor. When working at the right pace, the supervisor ensures that construction progresses smoothly, maintaining the structure's strength and stability. But if the supervisor pushes workers too hard without rest, the building process can become chaotic, leading to poor-quality construction and structural issues. Likewise, mTOR regulates growth and cell health when balanced, but if overactive, it can lead to problems like cancer and metabolic disorders.

This pathway works opposite of autophagy, which you learned in Chapter 2 is your body's cellular cleanup process and is more catabolic (in a good way). Protein requirements vary by age, gender, activity level, and health history, but a good rule of thumb is to consume at least 30 grams of protein at one meal to trigger the mTOR response. Your 30-Day Metabolic Freedom Reset will have a strong emphasis on these high-quality amino acids.

To achieve metabolic freedom, it's important to know which foods interfere with your metabolism and cause damage, such as high-fructose corn syrup, so that you can avoid them. The good news is that there are plenty of good fats, protein, fruits, vegetables, and fermented foods that are beneficial, delicious, and filling.

Now that you understand the right foods to support your hormones, gut, and metabolism, let's discuss the biggest piece of the metabolic puzzle: how your thoughts influence health or disease.

CHAPTER 10

HOW YOUR THOUGHTS INFLUENCE FAT LOSS AND HEALTH

A railroad employee was working late one night on the railroad tracks, and all of his co-workers had clocked out for the evening. This particular employee worked inside the refrigerator cart and didn't realize that it was past 11 P.M., and as he was getting ready to clock out himself, he found himself stuck inside the refrigerator cart. He banged on the door and shouted out for help to no avail. Everyone had gone home.

He started feeling cold and shivering. He tried to warm himself up but noticed he kept getting colder each hour. He began writing on the wall inside the railroad car, documenting his thoughts throughout the night. He wrote, "I'm stuck inside this car. It's freezing and all of my co-workers have gone home." As the hours passed, he kept glancing at the temperature apparatus inside the car, watching it plummet minute by minute. The next words he wrote were, "I'm getting colder and colder. The temperature is dropping rapidly." As more time passed, he started to think that he wasn't going to make it until the next morning at 7 A.M., when the next shift of employees came in.

The last words he wrote were, "I'm freezing to death. I'm not going to make it." When the next shift arrived in the morning, they opened up the car and found him dead. He had frozen to death. When they investigated the cause of death, it was from hypothermia. What was interesting was that during the investigation they determined that the temperature apparatus was broken. The temperature displayed was many degrees colder than the actual temperature in the car. The temperature never dropped below 55 degrees F, which is not low enough to cause hypothermia. This man's thoughts created the fact that he was freezing, and it manifested into his own demise. This cautionary tale shows how powerful the mind is.

Our thoughts have a direct influence on our health and longevity. Psychiatrists estimate that the average person has 60,000 thoughts every day. They also determined that 90 percent of those thoughts are the same thoughts from the day before, and 85 percent of those thoughts are negative. Motivational speaker and author Zig Ziglar called this stinkin' thinkin'. I believe if your thinkin' is stinkin', your health is shrinking!

In the book *Biology of Belief*, cell biologist Dr. Bruce Lipton made the case that thoughts are a frequency, and this frequency has the ability to penetrate your cell membrane and communicate with your DNA nucleus. If the thought is negative, the protein produced by your DNA is inflammatory. This shortens your telomeres and damages your DNA, leading to a shortened lifespan. If the thought is positive, the communication signal sent to your DNA produces anti-inflammatory proteins, which lengthen your telomeres and protect your DNA, extending your lifespan.

In this chapter we'll explore the placebo and nocebo effects and their influence on your health and wellness. You'll also learn the extraordinary power of gratitude and purpose as well as the impact your environment can have on your thoughts. If you have 60,000 thoughts per day, then you have 60,000 opportunities to place your entire body in a healing state, every single day. This is the greatest health biohack you will ever learn.

A Poor Self-Image Causes Weight-Loss Resistance

Allow me to share an idea that every human being should learn. Dr. Maxwell Maltz, author of *Psycho-Cybernetics*,[1] said in the 1960s that this was the greatest physiological discovery of his generation: Self-image directly influences our success. Let's say you have the self-image that you are an overweight person, and you make the decision to go on a diet and instantly move into action. You start to lose weight because you're cutting calories and possibly exercising more, but something happens a few weeks or months in: You find the weight you've lost. If you go on a diet without altering your self-image, any weight loss will be temporary. Because self-image is a cybernetic instrument, it measures the deviation from the set goal and immediately corrects course.

The autopilot system in an airplane is a prime example of how a cybernetic instrument operates. Imagine a plane taking off from Chicago with the destination set for Paris, France. Once the autopilot is engaged, it continuously monitors and adjusts the plane's course to ensure it stays on track to reach Paris. The pilot could, in theory, relax with the passengers, knowing the autopilot will correct any deviations from the intended path. Similarly, when someone has a self-image of being overweight, their internal cybernetic instrument—or subconscious mind—works to keep them aligned with that self-image. Even if they attempt to change their habits, they may find themselves gravitating back to unhealthy foods, like donuts and cookies, as their mind seeks to maintain the status quo of their overweight identity. Just as the autopilot course-corrects a plane, their self-image steers them back to behaviors that reinforce their existing beliefs about themselves. The weight that was lost is now found. To be successful, that person needs to change their self-image (paradigm) and release the weight. As Joel Barker says in *Paradigms: The Business of Discovering the Future,* "To be able to shape your future, you have to be willing and able to change your paradigm."[2]

How to Change a Paradigm

America's greatest prosperity teacher, Bob Proctor, explains that paradigms are a multitude of habits that guide every move you make. They affect the way you eat, the way you walk, even the way you talk. They govern your communication, your work habits, your successes, and your failures. There are only two ways to change the paradigm: an emotional impact or repetition.

Nine times out of ten an emotional impact will be a negative experience. For example, back in 2008 when I was going through a devastating breakup, feeling depressed and suicidal, it was enough of an emotional impact to change my paradigm. Eventually this resulted in me transforming my health. Another example of an emotional impact is a crisis like cancer or a serious car accident, when people are confronted with their mortality. Often this changes the way they think about themselves and their outlook on life. Again, it's usually a negative experience and not the ideal route.

Since significant emotional impacts are unpredictable, I strongly recommend using repetition, the second way to change a paradigm. Repetition is exposing yourself to a new idea over and over again. The point of this is not to memorize information, but rather to impress the idea or image into your subconscious or emotional mind enough times that it replaces the old idea or paradigm that resides there.

Affirmations are a great way to reinforce the new self-image. Part of your 30-Day Metabolic Freedom Reset will be to read the following affirmation each morning and before bed, when the subconscious mind is most impressionable: "I am so happy and grateful now that I am at my perfect weight. I am looking good, and I am feeling great. The perfect health I seek is now seeking me. I remove any blockages between us."

My client Claire is a powerful example of how mindset can shape our reality. In 2020, she was hospitalized with severe COVID-19, facing life-threatening complications, as her lungs failed and her oxygen levels plummeted. She endured several near-death experiences but eventually mustered the strength to pull through. After spending over a month in the hospital, Claire was released with a new lease on life. However, she was still over 40 pounds overweight and dealing with prediabetes, high blood pressure, and lingering long COVID symptoms that triggered multiple autoimmune conditions.

Claire often referred to herself as a "COVID survivor." I encouraged her to shift her perspective by writing down an affirmation, declaring herself a "COVID thriver" instead of merely a survivor. With this new self-image, she began making significant progress. Though she occasionally struggled with self-sabotage—her internal cybernetic instrument trying to course-correct to her old self-image—she used her affirmation as an anchor to break the cycle.

Over time, Claire reversed her prediabetes and high blood pressure. After years of relying on an oxygen tank nightly and while traveling, she recently received the green light to stop using it, as her lungs had recovered to optimal function. Her new self-image is one of someone who is thriving, not just surviving, and she continues to work on her health, inspiring her friends and family along the way. This transformation shows just how powerful a positive self-image can be when you fully embrace it.

The Placebo Effect

We've been told time after time that seeing is believing, but it actually works the opposite way. When we truly believe something, it will manifest to the point where we see it unfold before our eyes. Dr. Wayne Dyer emphasized the power of belief in shaping reality, encapsulated in his book *You'll See It When You Believe It.*

What prevents most people from achieving true metabolic health is their belief system, and because your environment impacts your belief system, it's important to protect your environment—from the people you spend time around to the commercials you watch and your social media feed. The placebo effect is a perfect example of this.

In his book *Anatomy of an Illness*, Dr. Norman Cousins explains how the placebo effect was discovered. It was during World War II, when an anesthesiologist named Dr. Henry Beecher ran out of morphine in the middle of a German bombardment.[3] Desperate to ease a soldier's pain, Beecher's nurse injected a syringe of saltwater but told the wounded man he was receiving the powerful painkiller. The soldier believed he was getting morphine. To Beecher's astonishment, the saline soothed the soldier's agony and kept him from going into shock. After Beecher returned to Harvard Medical School after the war, he pioneered the use of "controlled" clinical studies for new medicines, where some of the test subjects would unknowingly receive a placebo. By subtracting the improvement in the placebo control group, researchers could determine whether a drug really worked or not.

The Nocebo Effect

The placebo effect can work against you as well. This is called the "nocebo effect," and it's a neurobiological phenomenon that can cause negative outcomes when a patient has negative expectations about a treatment. We started this chapter with an example of this with the story of the railroad employee, but allow me to share another powerful illustration.

During a football game in Los Angeles several years ago, a few people became ill with symptoms of food poisoning. The doctor who treated them ascertained that they'd all had Coca-Cola from one of the two dispensing machines by the stands. He naturally wondered if the soda's syrup had been contaminated or the machines' copper piping had corroded. But before they could pinpoint the cause, he didn't want anyone else to be exposed, so he went on the public address system and described the symptoms of the sick people and warned everyone not to drink any more Coca-Cola.

Within minutes, the whole football stadium became full of vomiting people—including many who hadn't gone to either soda machine. There were five ambulances shuttling back and forth to bring people to a nearby hospital. Later that day, it was determined that there was nothing poisonous in the Coca-Cola machines. As soon as they received the news, the people in the hospital stopped throwing up. There was nothing wrong with them. Dr. Cousins called this "a mass-induced hypnosis," an acute physical reaction caused completely by people's minds.[4]

There's no question that fear can cause shortness of breath, our temperature to rise, and even make us vomit. Since we live in a world today where fear is the cultural standard, and we're supposed to avoid risk at all costs, most people let it take over their lives. But here's the reality: Life is risky. It's so risky, in fact, that none of us are going to get out of it alive! So it's critical that we learn to direct and control our own minds. Once we do this, we'll make ourselves not only healthier but happier as well, transforming the absolute quality of our lives. Bob Proctor nailed it when he said the following in his books *You Were Born Rich* and *The Art of Living*, "Faith and fear both demand for you to believe in something you cannot see; you choose!" In other words, "faith is the ability to see the invisible, believe in the incredible, and receive what the masses think is impossible."[5]

The Best Anti-Inflammatory Supplement in the World

One of the best ways to put yourself in a healing state—and rewire the brain to believe in healing at all—is with a supplement called vitamin G. Dr. Joe Dispenza is a neuroscientist, author, and lecturer known for his work on the intersection of science and spirituality, particularly how the brain and body can be reprogrammed through meditation and mental practices to achieve personal transformation and healing. He conducted a fascinating experiment where he took 120 people and measured their levels of cortisol and a chemical called IgA at the start and conclusion of the vitamin G workshop. As cortisol rises, IgA, which is a protein, one of the strongest building blocks of life, falls. IgA is responsible for the healthy function of our body's supreme internal defense system—the immune system. It's constantly fighting a barrage of bacteria, viruses, and organisms that invade and/or are already living within the body's internal environment. Bottom line: IgA is better than any flu shot or immune system booster we could possibly take—and it's totally natural.

During this four-day workshop, Dispenza asked 120 study participants to take vitamin G for nine to ten minutes, three times a day, to determine the following: If they could elevate their emotional states, could they also raise their immunity and reduce stress hormones like cortisol? He discovered at the conclusion of the event that the cortisol levels of participants dropped by three standard deviations, and their IgA levels shot up on average from 52.5 to 86. These are significant, measurable changes. He also observed that when vitamin G is taken, 1,200 different chemical reactions occur that begin to repair and restore the body.[6]

Another study published by the University of California, Davis, revealed that "People who take vitamin G have 16 percent lower diastolic blood pressure and 10 percent lower systolic blood pressure compared to those who take less vitamin G."[7] According to the same study, "People who take vitamin G have between 9 and 13 percent lower levels of hemoglobin A1c, a key marker of glucose control that plays a significant role in the diagnosis of diabetes."

Where can you purchase vitamin G? I don't have an affiliate link or coupon code, because vitamin G is the practice of gratitude. Yes, the studies I referenced are real, done on people who practice gratitude. Now we know that gratitude not only makes us feel good mentally and emotionally but also has a positive impact on our physical health.

How Gratitude Rewires Your Brain for Success

There's a part of your brain called the reticular activating system (RAS). It's the size of your pinky, located within the hypothalamus and brainstem. The job of the RAS is to regulate behavioral arousal, consciousness, and motivation. In simple terms, it was put inside your brain as a selective-seeking mechanism. There are millions of stimulations that the brain needs to filter out each day. The RAS is a software that we've trained to filter out what's not important, so we only see what is important. If we didn't have the RAS, the brain would short-circuit from too much stimulation.

Here's how it works in practical terms. Let's say you have a goal to purchase a new vehicle. You fall in love with a Tesla model Y, and your favorite color is red, so you begin researching red model Ys. You spend time online comparing new Teslas versus used Teslas, and leasing versus buying. After a few weeks of research, you decide to purchase a brand-new red Tesla. You purchase the car, drive it off the dealership lot, and notice something interesting. As you drive your new car, you begin to see the same exact car, a red Tesla, showing up all over your neighborhood. You notice red Teslas on the road, in parking lots, and at stoplights. Did everyone decide to buy a red Tesla because you purchased one? No, those red Teslas were always there, but now you've activated the RAS to see it!

In other words, if you feed energy into all of the problems you have in life—how unhealthy you are and the obstacles to getting well—you'll see more of this to verify your belief system. When you begin to feed energy into gratitude and healing, however, those obstacles become opportunities. This is a universal law: What you feed energy into expands. In other words, what you appreciate, appreciates. It's true that what you think about, and thank about, you bring about!

How Gratitude Improves Mitochondrial Health

Martin Picard, Ph.D., Associate Professor of Behavioral Medicine at Columbia University, and Elissa S. Epel, Ph.D., Professor in the Department of Psychiatry at the University of California, San Francisco, conducted a study on chronic stress and depleted mitochondrial function in caregivers.[8] This study looked at the functional index of mitochondrial health (MHI) for human leukocytes (immune cells that help the body fight infections and diseases). The MHI outperformed individual mitochondrial function measures, meaning the MHI was a very accurate way for assessing mitochondrial health. Elevated positive mood at night was associated with higher MHI, and nightly positive mood was also a mediator of the association between caregiving and MHI. In other words, when caregivers practiced gratitude at night, they had healthier mitochondria the next day. Moreover, MHI was correlated to positive mood on the days preceding, but not following, the blood draw, suggesting for the first time that mitochondria in humans may respond to proximate emotional states within days. Correspondingly, the caregiver group, which had higher perceived stress and lower positive and greater negative daily affect, exhibited lower MHI. This suggests that daily fluctuations in mood, especially toward more negative emotions, can adversely affect mitochondrial function over the course of a single day.

Do people who feel more positive and grateful have healthier mitochondria than those who feel negative? Is mitochondrial health shaping how we feel, or is it the other way around? The study revealed that morning and evening mood strongly predicted mitochondrial health, but mitochondrial health did not predict mood.

Vitamin G Extends Lifespan

Experiencing gratitude is linked to increased longevity in older women, according to a study published in *JAMA Psychiatry.*[9] Researchers from Harvard analyzed data from 49,275 older female nurses and found that higher levels of gratitude correlated with a 9 percent reduction in all-cause mortality and a 15 percent reduction in cardiovascular deaths. The study suggests that intentionally fostering gratitude, such as through regular gratitude journaling, can be a valuable psychological resource for promoting healthy aging and enhancing longevity.

The Health Benefits of Living on Purpose with Your Purpose

Robert Heinlein said, "In the absence of clearly defined goals, we become strangely loyal to performing daily trivia until ultimately we become enslaved by it."[10] Daily trivia can include numbing yourself with processed food, consuming social media, playing video games, and even drug abuse. I remember being enslaved by daily trivia in the form of video game addiction, drug addiction, and food addiction. I was told I had an "addictive personality," but I believe these bad behaviors were simply a result of not being clear on my highest values. Once I determined my purpose in life—which is to educate the world on metabolic health—and began to live on purpose with this purpose, I turned my addictions into a superpower.

Think about the amount of time and energy you spend on your own addictions. Once you become clear on your highest values, you can transfer this energy into a greater good, and it becomes a superpower. The word *obsession* typically has a negative connotation associated with it, but its definition is "an idea or thought that continually preoccupies or intrudes on a person's mind." If you become obsessed with your health goals, this is actually positive. Your obsessions become your possessions.

There's an area of study about your highest values called *telos*. This is a Greek term that refers to the ultimate aim, purpose, or goal of a person or thing. In philosophy, especially in Aristotle's works, telos signifies the inherent end that an object or being naturally seeks. For instance, the telos of an acorn is to become an oak tree. This concept is central to Aristotle's notion of causality and his ethical theory, where the telos of human life is to achieve eudaemonia, or flourishing and happiness. Understanding telos helps in comprehending why entities exist and behave in certain ways, emphasizing purpose-driven processes over random occurrences. Telos is also influential in ethical discussions, as it provides a framework for evaluating actions based on their contribution to achieving the highest good or ultimate purpose.

Lack of purpose is the leading cause of obesity and disease. In the groundbreaking book *Recovering the Soul*, Larry Dossey, M.D., shared a study that revealed that more heart attacks take place in the United States on Monday morning between 8 A.M. and 9 A.M. In other words, the majority of people have their first heart attack—85 percent of the American public, according to studies—going to jobs they hate. More recent studies support this.[11, 12] I believe we have an obesity crisis not necessarily because of what people are eating, but because of what's eating them.

When you're clear on your highest values, and live congruently with them, you become unstoppable. Obstacles turn into opportunities. You manifest the energy, health, and vitality to achieve your wildest dreams.

Why Finding Purpose after Retirement Is Essential for Health

Several studies have examined the relationship between retirement and increased mortality rates. Research from the National Bureau of Economic Research (NBER) found that male mortality rates increased by about 2 percent at age 62, coinciding with the eligibility for Social Security benefits, which often prompts a surge in retirements.[13] This study suggests that the lifestyle changes associated with retirement, such as reduced physical activity and social engagement, could contribute to this increase in mortality.

In 1978, Ellen Langer, a Harvard psychologist, conducted an important study,[14,15] in which she gave houseplants to two groups of nursing-home residents. One group was told they were responsible for keeping their plant alive, and that they had autonomy in their daily schedule; the other group was told that staff would care for their plant, and they were not given choices regarding their daily schedule. After 18 months, twice as many people in the group that was given responsibility for their plant and schedule were still alive as in the other group. Langer took this as evidence that the current biomedical model, which views the mind and body as separate, was wrong. In response, she conducted another study to examine further the mind's impact on the body.

In 1981, Langer and her graduate students transformed a building to mimic the year 1959, filling it with period-appropriate items like black-and-white TVs, old furniture, and magazines.16 Eight men over the age of 70 lived there for five days, instructed to act as if they were 22 years younger. They discussed 1950s events, watched old movies, and referred to themselves as they were in 1959. The men were treated as if they were in their 50s, not their 70s, and were not given any physical assistance, even when it was difficult. They were told to carry their belongings upstairs, one shirt at a time if necessary. This was to reinforce their younger self-image.

The goal was to see if mentally living in a younger era could trigger physical improvements. Remarkably, by the end of the study, the men showed improvements in hearing, eyesight, memory, dexterity, and appetite. Those who needed canes walked without them, and all participants displayed increased independence and vitality. Langer's experiment highlighted how changing perceptions of age and ability can lead to significant biological changes, offering the men an opportunity to view themselves not as elderly but as vibrant and capable individuals. This mental shift had profound physical effects, demonstrating the powerful connection between mind and body. Participants who maintained a youthful self-image by having clear goals and a sense of purpose in their lives experienced increased energy and vitality. This positive mindset and drive translated into healthier and fitter bodies as they worked toward achieving their objectives.

How Laughter Heals Your Body

Let's return to Dr. Norman Cousins, who was renowned for his pioneering work on the healing power of laughter. Diagnosed with a severe and painful condition called ankylosing spondylitis in the 1960s, Cousins was given a grim prognosis with little chance of recovery. However, he developed a unique approach to his treatment, emphasizing the therapeutic benefits of laughter and a positive attitude. Cousins found that watching comedic films like the Marx Brothers' movies and *Candid Camera* episodes significantly reduced his pain and improved his overall health. His regimen of "laugh therapy" included regular doses of humor, which he documented in his influential book *Anatomy of an Illness*.[17]

Cousins's experiences and subsequent research demonstrated that laughter could trigger the release of endorphins, the body's natural painkillers, and reduce stress hormones. This, in turn, enhanced immune function and promoted relaxation. His work has inspired further studies on the impact of humor and laughter on health, highlighting its potential to alleviate pain, improve cardiovascular health, and enhance emotional well-being. Overall, Norman Cousins's contributions have significantly shaped our understanding of the mind-body connection and the role of positive emotions in healing, making laughter an essential component of holistic health practices.

Incorporating laughter into daily routines may offer surprising benefits for metabolic health. Research has shown that participating in a structured laughter program can lead to measurable improvements in body composition, including reductions in body weight, BMI, and abdominal circumference. These effects are likely due to laughter's ability to reduce stress, a known contributor to metabolic dysfunction. Laughter has also been found to mimic the physiological benefits of moderate exercise by improving heart rate and muscle relaxation, further enhancing its potential to support metabolic health.[18]

Regular bouts of laughter can decrease levels of the stress hormone cortisol, which is often elevated in individuals with metabolic syndrome. By reducing cortisol and other stress-related biomarkers, laughter not only promotes a positive mental state but also contributes to a healthier metabolic profile. These findings suggest that incorporating more humor and laughter into your life could be a simple yet effective strategy to support metabolic health and overall well-being.[19]

Your Environment Determines Your Health

Environment is more important than heredity because it impacts the thoughts you think, your self-image, and your belief system. This determines the actions you take (or don't take), which then affect your results, and eventually your destiny.

I've noticed when I make changes in my life, my friends and family members are not always on board. This is because when someone changes, they become a threat to all those who don't. The perfect example of this is the "crabs in a bucket" story, which is often used to describe a situation where individuals in a group hold each other back from achieving success. It's similar to how crabs behave when trapped in a bucket: When one tries to escape, the others will pull it back down, ensuring that none of them escape. Similarly, some people may sabotage or discourage others' efforts to improve their circumstances out of envy, competition, or a desire to maintain the status quo.

This is why part of your 30-Day Metabolic Freedom Reset will be to do an environmental audit and to make the necessary changes for you to achieve massive success. This simple exercise will empower you to take control of your environment, which is crucial for mastering your metabolism. By engaging in this practice, you'll be able to clearly identify the people in your life who energize and support you versus those who drain your energy, often referred to as "crabs." Recognizing these influences is key to creating a positive, supportive atmosphere that fosters better metabolic health.

In my work with clients, I've come to see just how critical their thoughts and self-image are to their success. Even when someone is practicing keto and fasting and following the reset, if their mind still believes they'll never get healthy or lose the weight, they'll experience setbacks.

If you find yourself struggling at any point in the program, be sure to tune into your thoughts and make sure they are positive. In the next chapter I'll share some of my favorite cutting-edge health biohacks to make the process even smoother and easier for you.

CHAPTER 11

CUTTING-EDGE BIOHACKS TO ACHIEVE A NEW LEVEL OF HEALTH

Many people are fed up with the status quo, medical "sick care" system, and they're taking matters into their own hands by researching biohacks. *Biohacking* refers to the practice of making small, incremental lifestyle or dietary changes to improve health, well-being, and performance. It often involves using technology, supplements, and various self-experiments to optimize the body's functions.

I've been blessed to have interviewed more than 900 scientists, companies, and practitioners who research biohacking and longevity for my award-winning *Metabolic Freedom* podcast. This chapter is a synthesis of those interviews combined with my 17-plus years of research on this topic.

There are five key areas of biohacking that we will focus on in this chapter, so you can double your results in half the time:

1. supplements that biohack fat loss
2. biohacking wearables to track your progress
3. biohacking devices that lower inflammation and balance your nervous system

4. my favorite biohacks that utilize hormesis

5. free biohacks

Let's take the time to explore each of these now.

Supplements That Biohack Fat Loss

Not all supplements are created equal—in fact, many of the ones on the market result in expensive urine. The key is to use high-quality supplements derived from whole foods versus synthetic supplements made in a lab. When you take synthetic vitamins, the human body recognizes this substance as a drug. When you take real food supplements, the human body recognizes this as nutrition. What results is something called "selective absorption," wherein the body fills any nutritional gaps and excretes the rest. Real food supplements are derived from concentrated, dehydrated forms of fruits, vegetables, and other natural sources, providing a complex blend of vitamins, minerals, and phytonutrients as they occur in nature. To identify these supplements, look for labels that list whole foods like "organic spinach," "kale," "berries," or other recognizable plants as primary ingredients. Additionally, check for terms like "cold-pressed" or "raw" processing, which preserve nutrient integrity.

In contrast, synthetic supplements often list isolated nutrients, such as "ascorbic acid" for vitamin C or "dl-alpha-tocopherol" for vitamin E, indicating that these nutrients were manufactured in a lab rather than derived from a natural source. These products may lack the co-factors and other beneficial compounds found in whole foods that aid in nutrient absorption and efficacy. When selecting supplements, prioritize products that clearly state their whole foods origin, have minimal processing, and avoid fillers, additives, and artificial ingredients to ensure you're getting the best support for your health.

Here's a list of my favorite anti-inflammatory, fat-burning supplements to help you achieve metabolic freedom.

Coffee

For the purpose of this chapter, I will categorize coffee as a supplement. Coffee's most powerful polyphenol, chlorogenic acid (CGA), instructs your body's fat cells to burn their fatty acids for fuel. This is the same mechanism that statin drugs use to lower your cholesterol, without potential side effects. CGA cuts cravings, suppresses appetite, and activates the liver to produce more bile, aiding in detoxing your cells.

It helps the liver to process fats and glucose more efficiently by lowering triglyceride levels and stabilizing blood sugars. This blood sugar balancing act decreases your risk for metabolic syndrome and diabetes while inhibiting the growth of new fat cells. Studies suggest CGA reduces abdominal fat in overweight adults by working together with the caffeine in coffee to increase the number of cells that are burned for energy. It even works while you're sleeping![1]

CGA has been associated with antioxidant, antiviral, antibacterial, anticancer, and anti-inflammatory activity, as well as others that reduce the risk of cardiovascular diseases, type 2 diabetes, and Alzheimer's disease. However, the biological activities depend on the stability of CGAs, which are sensitive to pH, temperature, and light as well as individual differences in humans. We all have our own internal chemistry, biology, and functionality of our many glands, organs, and moving parts, and we metabolize CGA our own way and tolerate it differently.

The following points highlight decades of peer-reviewed scientific research about CGA:

- **It prevents cardiovascular disease.** Consuming high-CGA coffee may improve blood flow and endothelial function after meals, meaning chlorogenic acid may reduce some of the risk factors for cardiovascular disease and atherosclerosis.[2, 3]

- **It reduces inflammation.** Chlorogenic acid may help lower levels of inflammation and, over the long term, prevent chronic disease.[4]

- **It improves glucose regulation.** Having a diet rich in chlorogenic acid sources may help regulate glucose levels, which can be beneficial for losing weight and reducing the risk of diabetes.[5]

- **It lowers blood pressure.** Chlorogenic acid may benefit blood pressure by causing a statistically moderate reduction in diastolic and systolic blood pressure during the ingestion period.[6]

Choose an Organic Medium Roast

Caffeine is a well-researched ingredient known for its ability to boost metabolism and increase fat oxidation. Studies have shown that caffeine can enhance energy expenditure and promote weight loss by increasing the breakdown of fat and improving exercise performance.[7, 8]

Be sure to choose a medium roast as opposed to a dark one. Once the beans are roasted beyond medium, they've lost a whopping 75 percent of their fat-blasting polyphenols. Also, coffee grown in high altitudes with extreme temperature changes produces the most polyphenols. Make sure your coffee is organic and that it's been tested for contaminants such as mold, heavy metals, and pesticides. My personal favorite brands include Purity Coffee, Camano Island, Danger Coffee, Bulletproof, Lifeboost Coffee, and Regalo coffee.

Have a Coffee Curfew

It's a great idea to have a coffee curfew. The half-life of caffeine in the body varies widely depending on several factors, including age, body weight, pregnancy status, medication intake, and liver health. However, in most adults, the half-life is generally estimated to be between four and six hours.[9] This means that if you consume 100 milligrams of caffeine at 2 P.M., after four to six hours, which is around 6 to 8 P.M., 50 milligrams will remain in your system. After another four to six hours, or around 12 to 2 A.M., only 25 milligrams will remain, and so on. Some people, especially those sensitive to caffeine, may experience its effects for several hours or even days. It's best to have a coffee curfew of 10 A.M. to ensure it doesn't impact your quality of sleep.

The 90-Minute Caffeine Rule

As I mentioned earlier, waiting 90 minutes after waking up to have caffeine offers potential benefits like optimizing the natural rhythm of cortisol, a hormone promoting alertness. By delaying caffeine, your body utilizes this natural energy boost first, potentially leading to sustained energy and reduced caffeine reliance. Enhanced caffeine effectiveness is another benefit. Adenosine, a neurotransmitter promoting sleepiness, builds up while awake. Waiting 90 minutes allows adenosine levels to rise, making caffeine more effective in blocking its receptors, keeping you alert. It can also reduce caffeine dependency, as early morning consumption can lead to increased dependence, with your body relying less on natural cortisol. Delaying intake may help reduce this dependency and prevent potential withdrawal symptoms.

Improved sleep quality is also a potential benefit. Consuming caffeine too early can disrupt your sleep-wake cycle. Delaying intake may help improve your sleep quality by allowing your body to wind down naturally in the evening. Experiment to find what works best for you, paying attention to your body's response to caffeine at different times.

Caprylic Acid (C8) MCT Oil

MCT oil, particularly rich in caprylic acid, offers remarkable benefits for metabolism and mitochondrial uncoupling—which can be likened to a car engine running without engaging the gears. Normally, the engine (mitochondria) burns fuel (glucose or fat) to produce power (ATP) efficiently. In mitochondrial uncoupling, the fuel is still burned, but the energy is released as heat instead of storing energy as fat. This process dissipates energy and can increase metabolism, much like an idling car engine burns fuel without moving the car.

This mechanism can help in regulating body weight and protecting against metabolic diseases by increasing energy expenditure. Caprylic acid, a medium-chain triglyceride known for its health benefits, is rapidly absorbed and converted into ketones, providing a quick and efficient energy source. This process enhances metabolic rate and supports weight management. The dual action of boosting metabolism and enhancing mitochondrial function makes MCT oil a powerful ally in achieving optimal metabolic health. The medium-chain triglyceride caprylic acid shows the most promising research as it relates to these benefits.[10, 11, 12]

You can take MCT oil as a supplement or incorporate it into your diet through natural sources like coconut oil, sheep and goat dairy, butter, and ghee. These foods provide a convenient and natural way to boost your intake of MCTs, including caprylic acid.

Vinegar and Apple Cider Vinegar (ACV)

There's a ton of research showing apple cider vinegar boosts metabolism, suppresses appetite, and reduces fat storage. It has three major benefits:

1. **Weight loss:** ACV contains acetic acid, which has been shown to ramp up metabolism, curb cravings by up to 600 calories per day, and inhibit fat storage. This also helps people lose weight even when they're having trouble.

2. **Digestion:** Most of us are nutrient deficient to some degree and suffer from some level of gut dysfunction. Because ACV is so acidic, it can help restore stomach acidity, prevent heartburn, aid protein digestion, assist bile/enzyme release, and so much more.

3. **Blood sugar stabilization:** ACV has been shown in numerous studies to mitigate blood sugar spikes in people with normal blood sugar, prediabetics, and even diabetics. It can also help reduce sugar spikes (even with foods like bread), which can be difficult for people to avoid.

One study investigated the effects of vinegar supplementation on glucose and insulin responses and satiety after a meal of white bread. Twelve healthy volunteers consumed bread with varying amounts of vinegar. Results showed a significant dose-response relationship; higher vinegar levels led to lower glucose and insulin responses and increased satiety. The study suggests that vinegar can reduce blood glucose and insulin levels after meals while increasing feelings of fullness, indicating potential benefits for dietary management.[13]

Another study titled "Vinegar Intake Reduces Body Weight, Body Fat Mass, and Serum Triglyceride Levels in Obese Japanese Subjects" examined the effects of vinegar on obesity. In a 12-week, double-blind trial, obese participants were given drinks with either 0, 15, or 30 milliliters of vinegar. Results showed significant reductions in body weight, BMI, visceral fat area, waist circumference, and serum triglyceride levels in the vinegar groups compared to the placebo group. This suggests that daily vinegar intake could help prevent metabolic syndrome by reducing obesity.[14]

THE THREE BEST TIMES TO USE VINEGAR OR ACV FOR OPTIMAL FAT LOSS

- **Fifteen to 20 minutes before your next meal:** Take 3 capsules (or 1 tablespoon diluted with water) before your next meal to improve digestion and mitigate blood sugar surges. This is one of the best ways to balance blood sugars.

- **After your meal:** Taking vinegar or ACV after your meal can do wonders if you experience bloating, gas, or have more carbs than you may have been expecting to consume. This can also assist in post-meal glucose levels. A study showed ACV improved insulin sensitivity after a high-carb meal up to 34 percent.[15] Bonus points if you go for a 15-minute walk too!

- **First thing in the morning:** Set yourself up for daily success by reducing cravings throughout the day, which can help you push further into your fast.

African Mango

African mango (Irvingia gabonensis) can promote weight loss, especially around your waist and hips. One of the most significant studies on it for fat loss in humans is a systematic review that analyzed several clinical trials: This review found that African mango extract significantly reduced body weight, body fat percentage, and waist circumference over periods of 4 to 10 weeks. In the most notable clinical trial, 102 overweight volunteers were given 150 milligrams of the extract twice daily before meals for 10 weeks, resulting in an average weight loss of 13 kilograms, a decrease in waist size by 16 centimeters, and improvements in cholesterol and blood glucose levels.[16, 17]

Another study on African mango showed significant reduction in body weight, body fat, and waist circumference in overweight humans in a randomized, double-blind, placebo-controlled investigation. It was also found to improve metabolic parameters, such as total cholesterol, LDL cholesterol, blood glucose, C-reactive protein, adiponectin, and leptin levels in overweight and obese participants.[18]

L-Carnitine

L-carnitine, a naturally occurring amino acid derivative, is widely recognized for its potential fat-loss and health benefits. It plays a crucial role in energy production by transporting long-chain fatty acids into the mitochondria, where they are oxidized to produce energy. This process helps in reducing body fat, enhancing exercise performance, and increasing muscle mass. Studies have shown that L-carnitine supplementation can improve fat metabolism, particularly during physical activity, leading to more effective weight loss.

Additionally, L-carnitine has been linked to improved heart health, reduced muscle soreness, and enhanced recovery after exercise. One of the most comprehensive studies on L-carnitine for fat loss was conducted by researchers at the National Institutes of Health (NIH). This 12-week study involved participants taking L-carnitine supplements along with a high-carbohydrate beverage twice a day. The participants also engaged in 30 minutes of low-intensity exercise such as walking or jogging four days a week. The study found that those on L-carnitine supplementation burned more calories during exercise, had increased muscle carnitine levels, and maintained their weight, while the non-L-carnitine group gained weight and had reduced calorie burn. These results suggest that L-carnitine can enhance fat metabolism and support weight loss when combined with regular exercise and proper diet.[19, 20, 21]

You can get L-carnitine in supplement form and from food. The top five foods rich in carnitine are:

1. beef steak (56 to 162 mg per 4-ounce serving)

2. ground beef (65 to 74 mg per 3-ounce serving)

3. pork meat (20 to 30 mg per 3-ounce serving)

4. whole milk (8 mg per 8 ounces)

5. codfish (3 to 5 mg per 3-ounce serving)

Green Tea Leaf Extract

Green tea leaf extract, rich in antioxidants like epigallocatechin gallate (EGCG), has been widely studied for its health and fat-loss benefits. EGCG helps boost metabolism and increase fat oxidation, particularly during exercise. Studies have shown that green tea extract can enhance thermogenesis, the body's process of burning calories to produce heat, which contributes to weight loss and improved body composition. Additionally, green tea extract has been linked to reduced appetite and improved fat distribution, making it an effective supplement for weight management. Beyond weight loss, green tea extract offers health benefits, such as improved heart health, better blood sugar regulation, and reduced risk of certain cancers due to its high antioxidant content.

Research in the *International Journal of Obesity* revealed that green tea extract significantly increased energy expenditure and fat oxidation in humans.[22] The catechins found in green tea have the potential to target belly fat, especially in overweight and obese adults. Catechins are a type of natural phenol and antioxidant that belong to the flavonoid family, and are highly regarded for their potential health benefits. A study from the *Journal of Nutrition* evaluated the influence of a green tea catechin beverage on body composition and fat distribution in overweight and obese adults during exercise-induced weight loss. Participants were randomly assigned to receive a beverage containing 625 milligrams of catechins with 39 milligrams of caffeine or a control beverage (39 milligrams caffeine, no catechins) for 12 weeks, and they were asked to maintain constant energy intake and engage in ≥180 minutes/week of moderate intensity exercise, including ≥3 supervised sessions per week. At the end of the 12 weeks, researchers found that the green tea catechin consumption group achieved enhanced exercise-induced changes in abdominal fat and serum triglycerides.[23]

Forskolin Extract

Forskolin extract, derived from the root of the *Coleus forskohlii* plant, has been studied for its potential benefits in fat loss and weight management. Forskolin is known to stimulate the production of cyclic adenosine monophosphate (cAMP), a molecule that plays a crucial role in regulating metabolism and energy production. By increasing cAMP levels, forskolin can enhance the breakdown of stored fats and boost fat oxidation.

Research indicates that forskolin may help reduce body fat percentage and increase lean body mass, making it a promising supplement for improving body composition. One of the most notable studies on this was conducted at Baylor University and published in the journal *Obesity Research*. This randomized, double-blind, placebo-controlled study involved 30 overweight and obese men who were given 250 milligrams of a 10 percent forskolin extract twice daily for 12 weeks. The results showed that the forskolin group experienced a significant reduction in body fat percentage and an increase in lean body mass compared to the placebo group. Additionally, the forskolin group had higher testosterone levels, which may have contributed to the fat loss and muscle mass retention observed during the study.[24]

Grains of Paradise

One of the most notable studies on the effectiveness of grains of paradise (Aframomum melegueta) for fat loss in humans was published in the *Journal of Nutritional Science and Vitaminology*. This study involved 19 non-obese female volunteers who took 30 milligrams of grains of paradise extract daily for four weeks. The results showed a significant increase in whole-body energy expenditure and a reduction in visceral fat. The study concluded that grains of paradise extract could be a safe and effective method for reducing body fat, primarily by preventing the accumulation of visceral fat.[25] Another double-blind, placebo-controlled study involving 70 men and women also showed that supplementation with grains of paradise resulted in significant weight loss by increasing energy expenditure and reducing visceral fat.[26]

A significant study published in the *British Journal of Nutrition* focused on the effects of grains of paradise on brown adipose tissue (BAT) and energy expenditure. This study involved 19 healthy male volunteers who took an ethanolic extract of grains of paradise. The results indicated that the extract increased energy expenditure through the activation of BAT, which is responsible for thermogenesis and burning calories.[27]

Garcinia Cambogia

Garcinia cambogia, a tropical fruit also known as Malabar tamarind, has gained attention for its potential weight-loss benefits. The active ingredient in the fruit's rind, hydroxycitric acid (HCA), is believed to help inhibit the enzyme ATP citrate lyase, which the body uses to make fat. By blocking this enzyme, HCA is thought to prevent fat storage and reduce appetite by increasing serotonin levels in the brain, which can lead to reduced cravings and emotional eating. Some studies suggest that Garcinia cambogia can also enhance fat metabolism and increase exercise endurance, making it a popular supplement for those seeking to manage their weight. A meta-analysis in the *Journal of Obesity* reviewed multiple trials and concluded that Garcinia cambogia extract can result in short-term weight loss.[28]

Conjugated Linoleic Acid

Conjugated linoleic acid (CLA) is a type of polyunsaturated fatty acid that has been studied for its potential health benefits, particularly in the context of weight loss and fat reduction. Research suggests that CLA may help reduce body fat by inhibiting the storage of fat and promoting the breakdown of existing fat stores. Additionally, CLA is believed to increase energy expenditure and improve lean body mass, making it beneficial for those looking to enhance body composition. The *Journal of Nutrition* published a study showing that CLA supplementation led to a reduction in body fat mass in overweight and obese individuals.[29] Additional studies also revealed the benefit of CLA for fat loss.[30, 31]

You can get CLA from a supplement, but it is also found naturally in meat and dairy products such as heavy cream, butter, ghee, cottage cheese, sheep dairy, and cow cheese.

Capsaicin

Capsaicin, the active component in chili peppers, is renowned for its thermogenic properties and potential benefits for fat loss. Capsaicin works by activating the transient receptor potential vanilloid 1 (TRPV1), which increases the body's heat production and energy expenditure—this thermogenic effect can enhance fat oxidation and boost metabolism. Studies have demonstrated that capsaicin can significantly reduce abdominal fat and overall body fat by increasing calorie burn and promoting the breakdown of fat. Additionally, it has been shown to suppress appetite, leading to reduced calorie intake and supporting weight-loss efforts. A study in the *European*

Journal of Nutrition highlighted that capsaicin intake increased thermogenesis and fat oxidation, contributing to body fat reduction.[32]

Melatonin

Most people think of melatonin as merely a sleep supplement, but research reveals that its benefits extend far beyond sleep. In fact, melatonin plays a significant role in metabolism. As we know, healthy mitochondria are crucial for fat loss and longevity, and melatonin is the most potent antioxidant for these cellular powerhouses. Every cell in your body, except red blood cells, contains mitochondria, and these mitochondria produce their own melatonin.

One unique aspect of melatonin is that it doesn't have a negative feedback loop. This means you can supplement with high doses of it for extended periods, and your body will continue to produce it naturally. This is unlike other hormones, such as testosterone, where external supplementation can reduce the body's own production.

In his book *Melatonin: Miracle Molecule,* Dr. John Lieurance explores the extensive benefits of melatonin beyond its well-known role in regulating sleep.[33] He delves into how melatonin's powerful anti-inflammatory properties help reduce chronic inflammation, a key factor in many diseases. Additionally, it promotes fat loss by enhancing mitochondrial function and increasing metabolic rate. Dr. Lieurance also highlights melatonin's role in supporting longevity by protecting cellular health and reducing oxidative stress. His comprehensive guide reveals how high-dose melatonin can be a pivotal element in achieving optimal health and extending lifespan.

Dr. John Lieurance, who's a good friend of mine, wrote the following passage on melatonin, specifically for this book:

> Melatonin is often misunderstood as merely a sleep hormone, but it is, in fact, the ultimate resilience molecule, providing support at the cellular level, particularly during times of stress. While stress is commonly perceived as a mental or emotional burden, the most fundamental form of stress is inflammation. Melatonin has been largely confined to the role of a sleep aid by the current medical establishment, overshadowing its broader benefits. Unfortunately, this focus on pharmaceuticals often leads to the neglect of powerful, natural alternatives like melatonin, which can be incredibly effective and accessible.
>
> Is melatonin just for sleep? The truth is that melatonin is produced in every cell of your body. It is particularly concentrated in the gut, where its levels are 400 percent higher than elsewhere, supporting beneficial flora through a process known as *microbiome swarming*. In the brain's neurons and heart muscles,

melatonin protects these vital tissues from damage. It plays a crucial role in maintaining optimal cellular energy production, ensuring that your cells operate efficiently even under stress.

When cellular stress becomes too intense, the mitochondria—the energy powerhouses of the cell—shut down, forcing the cell to produce energy through a less efficient process called fermentation. This switch, known as the Warburg effect, is part of the body's attempt to adapt to stress, a phenomenon recently described as the "cell danger response." But how does melatonin fit into this picture? As a premier antioxidant, melatonin neutralizes the by-products of oxygen metabolism, preventing the cellular damage and degeneration that lead to conditions like infections, toxicity, atherosclerosis, and even aging. Studies have demonstrated that administering melatonin exogenously can reboot the body's systems during periods of extreme stress. For example, research has shown that melatonin can dramatically increase survival rates against some of the deadliest microbes known to humanity.[34]

What about COVID-19? Studies have shown that melatonin can be an effective treatment for COVID-19, not only reducing the risk of death but also lowering the transmission rate by 54 percent.[35, 36]

Supplementing with melatonin is safe, even at higher doses. Extensive research has shown no negative effects, even at doses equivalent to 150,000 mg for an average adult. Since melatonin does not create a negative feedback loop, its benefits are significant, and the risks are minimal or nonexistent. I've found that melatonin delivery via suppositories, such as MitoZen's Sandman, is particularly effective due to the poor oral bioavailability of melatonin—only about 2.5 percent of orally ingested melatonin makes it into the bloodstream. I've personally witnessed remarkable benefits from high-dose melatonin, both in myself and in my patients, some of whom I regularly prescribe doses of 200 mg or more.

In conclusion, melatonin is nothing to fear. On the contrary, it can be a powerful ally in our modern world, where we are bombarded by stressors that can shut down our cellular energy production. Without proper adaptation to these stressors, disease is likely to follow. To age gracefully, consider making melatonin a part of your nightly routine, especially after the age of 40 or 50.

The study "Is Melatonin the 'Next Vitamin D'?" reviews the expanding understanding of melatonin's functions beyond sleep regulation. It highlights melatonin's antioxidant properties, its role in immune function, and its influence on mitochondrial health, comparing it to vitamin D in terms of its wide-ranging health effects.

The study suggests that melatonin could be as significant as vitamin D in maintaining overall health.[37]

Biohacking Wearables to Track Your Progress

We live in an amazing world, where we have more access to information from our phones than the President of the United States had just 30 years ago. As the field of biohacking continues to become more popular, more devices to track our metabolic progress have flooded the market. In this section, I'll outline the best biohacking wearables to include on your 30-Day Metabolic Freedom Reset. These are not required for your reset to be successful, but they will help you achieve faster results if you decide to use any of them. Feel free to choose any of the following devices that resonate with you the most.

Continuous Glucose Monitor (CGM)

This is a revolutionary tool in the management of metabolic health, offering real-time insights into blood glucose levels. Unlike traditional glucose monitoring, which typically involves periodic finger-stick tests, a CGM continuously tracks glucose levels throughout the day and night via a small sensor inserted under the skin. A continuous glucose monitor (CGM) is applied by attaching a small sensor to the skin, typically on the abdomen or upper arm, which measures glucose levels in the interstitial fluid through a tiny filament inserted just beneath the skin. This technology provides dynamic glucose readings every few minutes, allowing individuals to see how their glucose levels respond to food, exercise, stress, and sleep in real time.

The benefits of using a CGM extend beyond mere convenience; it empowers users with the data needed to make informed lifestyle and dietary choices, helps in identifying glucose trends and patterns, and can significantly improve glycemic control. Moreover, CGMs can alert users to dangerous highs and lows in blood sugar levels, thereby preventing potential health crises. As a result, CGMs are not only invaluable for individuals managing diabetes but also for those looking to optimize their overall metabolic health and prevent the onset of metabolic diseases.

Sleep Trackers

In the realm of optimizing metabolic health, wearable sleep trackers like the Oura Ring and WHOOP band provide comprehensive insights into sleep quality, duration, and patterns, offering a detailed analysis of the different stages of sleep—deep, light, and REM. The Oura Ring, for instance, tracks a range of physiological signals, including heart rate variability, body temperature, and respiratory rate, to deliver a nuanced picture of overall sleep health. Similarly, the Whoop band excels in monitoring not only sleep but also recovery and strain, giving users a holistic view of how their daily activities impact their nightly rest.

The benefits of using sleep trackers extend beyond mere sleep monitoring. By providing actionable data, these devices empower users to make informed decisions about their lifestyle, from adjusting bedtime routines to optimizing physical activity levels. The insights gleaned from these trackers can lead to improved sleep hygiene, better recovery, enhanced athletic performance, and overall well-being. Additionally, by highlighting trends and deviations in sleep patterns, these devices can alert users to potential health issues early, allowing for timely interventions. In the context of metabolic health, quality sleep is crucial, as poor sleep is linked to insulin resistance, weight gain, and a host of other metabolic disorders. Thus, integrating sleep trackers into your health regimen can be a game-changer for achieving and maintaining optimal metabolic health.

STRATEGIES TO GET
BETTER SLEEP STARTING TONIGHT

Cool Your Room: Set the temperature to 60 to 68°F. This cool range helps lower your core body temperature, which signals your body to sleep. Consider a cooling mattress pad for temperature control.

Limit Electronics: Power down all devices an hour before bed. Light and stimulation from screens delay melatonin release and can elevate your heart rate, making it harder to unwind.

Eliminate Light: Block all sources of light to promote melatonin production, essential for restful sleep and overall health. Dark curtains or sleep masks can make a big difference.

Stop Eating at Least 3 Hours before Bed: Avoiding food at least 3 hours before bed improves sleep by allowing your body to focus on rest and recovery, rather than digestion, which can interfere with deep, restorative sleep.

> **Leverage the "Money Time Sleep Window:** Sleep between 10:00 P.M. and 2:00 A.M. for maximum restorative benefits. This period aligns with your circadian rhythm and is known to double the value of each hour of sleep.
>
> **Get Morning and Evening Sunlight Through Your Eyes:** Morning sunlight helps regulate your circadian rhythm by signaling wakefulness, while evening sunlight aids in winding down, both supporting deeper, more restful sleep.

Biohacking Devices That Lower Inflammation and Balance Your Nervous System

Inflammation and stress wreak havoc on your metabolic health, so some biohacking devices use sounds, visualizations, and vibrations to calm your body, reduce stress, and help you enter deeper states of relaxation. They promote better sleep and improve overall mental health and wellness by helping to regulate the autonomic nervous system, thereby reducing stress and promoting a state of equilibrium between the sympathetic (fight-or-flight) and parasympathetic (rest-and-digest) responses. The following devices achieve this and much more.

BrainTap

This innovative tool is designed to enhance mental health and cognitive performance through the use of brain wave entrainment. It combines sound and light therapy to synchronize brain waves. Users typically wear a headset that delivers these stimuli to the auditory and visual pathways, guiding the brain into specific states associated with deep relaxation, improved focus, and better cognitive function.

One of the primary benefits of BrainTap is its ability to reduce stress. The system uses guided visualization and soothing audio to help users enter a state of deep relaxation, which can significantly lower stress levels and promote overall mental well-being. Additionally, BrainTap can improve sleep quality by helping users achieve a state of relaxation before bedtime, which is essential for restorative sleep.

The device is also useful for enhancing cognitive performance: regular use can lead to improved focus and mental clarity, making it a valuable tool for individuals looking to optimize their mental performance, whether for work, study, or personal development. By integrating BrainTap sessions into daily routines, users can experience long-term benefits such as reduced anxiety, better emotional control, and enhanced mental resilience.

The inHarmony Meditation Cushion

This cushion is a versatile and innovative tool designed to enhance your meditation practice through the power of vibroacoustic therapy. Launched in 2020, it uses sound and music vibrations to penetrate your body, helping you achieve deeper, faster, and longer meditative states. By integrating vibroacoustics, the cushion creates an immersive musical experience that can make meditation more enjoyable and maintainable, promoting relaxation and reducing stress and anxiety quickly.

The cushion connects users to a supportive community via the inHarmony app, which provides access to guided meditations, chanting, breathwork, and educational talks in real time, led by professionals. The cushion is made from eco-friendly materials and is designed for comfort and portability. It is suitable for various settings, including home, office, and travel, making it a practical choice for those looking to enhance their mindfulness practices. Users have reported benefits like increased focus, mental clarity, improved mood, and reduced muscle recovery time. The inHarmony Meditation Cushion also supports proper posture and alignment, which can alleviate discomfort during long meditation sessions.

Apollo Neuro

A groundbreaking wearable device, the Apollo Neuro was designed to improve resilience to stress by delivering gentle vibrations to the body, which stimulate the parasympathetic nervous system. Worn on the wrist or ankle, Apollo Neuro leverages scientifically proven touch therapy to help users manage stress, enhance focus, and improve sleep quality. These vibrations mimic natural rhythms, which can help to shift the body from a fight-or-flight state to a rest-and-digest state, promoting a sense of calm and well-being. Studies have shown that regular use of Apollo Neuro can lead to significant reductions in stress and anxiety levels, improved heart rate variability, and better sleep patterns, all of which are crucial for maintaining metabolic health. By incorporating Apollo Neuro into daily routines, users can better manage their stress responses, thereby supporting overall metabolic function and well-being.

My Favorite Biohacks That Utilize Hormesis

As we discussed, hormesis is a stress you apply that forces your cells to adapt. This adaptation creates healthier cells, less inflammation, and more resiliency. The biohacks in this section use red and near-infrared light, hot and cold therapy, and electromagnetic pulses to stimulate hormesis for better metabolic health and fat loss.

Red Light Therapy (RLT)

RLT devices have emerged as a revolutionary tool in the realm of metabolic health, offering a noninvasive, science-backed method to enhance cellular function and promote overall well-being. These devices can be used for light exposure in regulating circadian rhythms and boosting metabolic processes.

RLT operates by emitting wavelengths of red and near-infrared light that penetrate the skin, stimulating mitochondrial function—the powerhouse of our cells. This enhancement in mitochondrial activity accelerates energy production, aids in tissue repair, and reduces inflammation, all crucial for optimal metabolic function. Moreover, consistent use of red light therapy has been shown to improve insulin sensitivity, support weight loss, and enhance muscle recovery, making it an invaluable addition to any metabolic health regimen. Adding RLT to daily routines can serve as a pivotal strategy for combating metabolic disorders and promoting long-term health vitality. The optimal dosage seems to be 10 minutes, twice per day.

Much research has been conducted on the use of RLT. For example, a comprehensive review paper summarized a vast amount of research on the effects of red and near-infrared light therapy on skin health. It covered various applications—including wound healing, anti-aging, and treatment of skin conditions like acne and psoriasis—and highlighted the positive effects of RLT on collagen production, inflammation reduction, and overall skin rejuvenation.[38]

Then there was a study that explored the cellular and molecular mechanisms behind RLT, focusing on its impact on mitochondria—it explained how red light therapy can enhance mitochondrial function, leading to improved cellular energy production, reduced oxidative stress, and enhanced tissue repair. This research provides valuable insights into the fundamental processes underlying the therapeutic effects of RLT.[39]

Another study investigated the effects of RLT on abdominal fat in overweight individuals. Participants who received RLT treatments experienced a significant reduction in waist circumference compared to the control group. This study suggests that RLT may help target localized fat deposits and promote body contouring.[40]

Finally, a randomized controlled trial examined the impact of RLT on body measurements in individuals seeking noninvasive body contouring. The study found that participants who received RLT treatments experienced significant reductions in waist, hip, and thigh circumferences compared to the control group, adding further support to the potential of RLT for reducing body fat and improving body shape.[41]

Choosing a Red Light Therapy Device

Choosing the right RLT device can be overwhelming, but understanding the science behind wavelengths can help you make an informed decision. Here are some tips:

1. **Focus on effective wavelengths:** Research indicates that red light (620 to 700 nm) and near-infrared (NIR) light (780 to 850 nm) are the most effective wavelengths for therapeutic benefits. Red light mainly targets the skin, promoting collagen production, reducing inflammation, and improving skin conditions. NIR light penetrates deeper, potentially enhancing muscle recovery, reducing pain, and improving cellular function.

2. **Consider your goals:** Devices with red light wavelengths (630 nm, 660 nm) are ideal for addressing skin concerns like wrinkles, acne, and wound healing. NIR wavelengths (810 nm, 830 nm, 850 nm) are more effective for deeper tissue penetration, potentially aiding in pain management, inflammation reduction, and muscle recovery. Devices that offer a combination of red and NIR wavelengths can provide a broader range of benefits for both skin and deeper tissues.

3. **Check device specifications:** Ensure the device clearly lists the wavelengths it emits and the power output (measured in milliwatts or mW). Higher power output generally means deeper penetration and potentially faster results.

The brands I personally use for red light devices include Bon Charge, SaunaSpace, Joovv, and Mito Red Light. You can also find red light devices at many spas, gyms, dermatology clinics, and chiropractic offices.

Cold Exposure

A potent tool for enhancing metabolic health, this therapeutic approach involves exposing the body to cold temperatures through methods like ice baths, cold plunges, cryotherapy, or cold showers. You can find cryotherapy devices and cold plunges at wellness centers, spas, sports medicine clinics, and chiropractic offices. The primary benefit of cold therapy lies in its ability to stimulate brown fat activation. Unlike white fat, which stores energy, brown fat burns calories to generate heat, thereby boosting metabolism. This process of thermogenesis can lead to improved fat loss and better weight management, and it's considered a promising target in the fight against the obesity epidemic.

The biggest activator of brown fat is moderate cold exposure. One study found that people with brown fat burned more calories. As Dr. Florian W. Kiefer, one of the study's authors, explained, "This data improves our understanding of how brown fat works in humans. We found that individuals with active brown fat burned 20 more kilocalories than those without."[42]

Additionally, cold exposure triggers a significant release of epinephrine (adrenaline) and norepinephrine (noradrenaline) in the brain and body. These neurochemicals make you feel alert and focused. Cold causes their levels to remain elevated for some time, and their ongoing effect after the exposure is to increase your level of energy and focus, which can help you have a more productive day.[43, 44]

Furthermore, the increased norepinephrine levels induced by cold exposure have been linked to various potential benefits, including:

- **Enhanced mood:** Norepinephrine is involved in mood regulation, and its release can contribute to feelings of well-being and euphoria.

- **Improved metabolism:** Norepinephrine can stimulate brown fat activity, which can increase energy expenditure and potentially aid in weight management.[45]

- **Pain relief:** Norepinephrine can have analgesic effects by activating descending pain inhibitory pathways.

Regular cold therapy sessions can also reduce inflammation, accelerate muscle recovery, and enhance overall immune function. Research led by Dr. Andrew Huberman and others indicates that accumulating 11 minutes of cold exposure per week can provide significant health benefits. This protocol involves short sessions of 1 to 5 minutes spread across two to four days.

A recent study suggests that cold exposure in the morning is better than later in the day. The study discusses how it shows a diurnal variation and unfolds differently in men and women. In men, cold-induced thermogenesis is higher in the morning than in the evening. Women experience no difference in cold-induced thermogenesis between morning and evening; however, their lipid metabolism is more modulated in the morning. The study suggests that brown adipose tissue activity may be higher in the morning in both sexes.[46]

Several studies suggest that pre-cooling (cold exposure) before exercise, especially in hot environments, can improve endurance performance, reduce perceived exertion, and potentially enhance power output.[47, 48] I personally think it's a good idea to engage in cold exposure before exercise and not after, since exercise naturally produces a healthy inflammatory response, and cold exposure after exercise may blunt your innate intelligence's ability to respond to the stress of exercise. This is also why taking a handful of antioxidant supplements after exercise is not a good idea.

Heat Therapy

A staple in the tool kit of metabolic health, heat therapy leverages the power of elevated temperatures to promote a multitude of health benefits. By exposing the body to heat through methods such as saunas, hot baths, or infrared therapy, heat therapy induces a state of hyperthermia that triggers a range of physiological responses. One of the primary benefits is the enhancement of circulation, as heat causes blood vessels to dilate, improving blood flow and delivering more oxygen and nutrients to tissues. This improved circulation aids in muscle recovery, reduces stiffness, and alleviates pain, making it particularly beneficial for those with chronic conditions such as arthritis.[49, 50]

Heat therapy stimulates the release of heat shock proteins, which play a critical role in protecting cells from stress and promoting cellular repair. This process can enhance overall metabolic function and resilience. There are also detoxification benefits of heat therapy, as sweating helps to eliminate toxins from the body, supporting liver function and improving skin health. Additionally, regular use of heat therapy has been linked to improved cardiovascular health, reduced inflammation, and enhanced immune function. Incorporating heat therapy into a holistic approach to metabolic health can thus provide a comprehensive boost to physical and mental well-being, promoting longevity and vitality.[51, 52, 53]

Regular sauna use has been shown to improve cardiovascular health by increasing heart rate and improving circulation, similar to the effects of moderate exercise. This can lead to better blood pressure management, enhanced cardiovascular fitness, and a reduction in the risk of heart disease and stroke. Studies have found that those who use a sauna two to three times per week have a 12 percent reduction in stroke risk, which increases to 62 percent for those who use it four to seven times per week.[54, 55]

For optimal results, use the sauna in a semi-fasted state and ensure proper hydration before and after sessions. Research indicates that spending around 20 minutes per session in a sauna, totaling about 60 to 90 minutes per week, can provide the significant health benefits outlined above. This time can be broken into multiple sessions, typically two to three times per week, each lasting 15 to 20 minutes. You can find different types of saunas at spa and wellness facilities, fitness centers, hotels and resorts, and health clubs.

Pulsed Electromagnetic Field (PEMF) Mats

PEMF mats have gained recognition in the field of metabolic health for their ability to enhance cellular function and promote overall well-being. The noninvasive nature of PEMF therapy, which utilizes electromagnetic fields to stimulate and rejuvenate cells, operates by emitting pulses that penetrate deep into the body, energizing cells and enhancing their repair processes.

One of the primary benefits of PEMF mats is the improvement of circulation, which facilitates better nutrient and oxygen delivery to tissues, aiding in recovery and reducing inflammation. PEMF therapy has also been shown to enhance cellular metabolism by improving the function of the mitochondria, which can lead to increased energy levels, better sleep, and a reduction in pain and stiffness. PEMF mats support bone health by stimulating osteoblasts, which are crucial for bone formation and repair.

Free Biohacks

Some of the best biohacks we have available to us are completely free. They might not be as sexy as an infrared sauna or red light therapy devices, but they can be just as effective.

Grounding/Earthing

Grounding, also known as earthing, involves direct contact with Earth's surface, such as walking barefoot or using conductive devices (ground mats and sheets). You see, Earth's surface holds a natural negative charge, primarily generated by lightning strikes and the planet's molten core. This negative charge is abundant in free electrons, which are constantly replenished, and when we make direct contact with the earth, these free electrons can transfer into our bodies.[56]

Our modern lifestyle, with its abundance of electronics and insulation from the ground, tends to create a positive charge buildup within us. This positive charge is associated with free radicals, unstable molecules that can damage cells and contribute to inflammation. The influx of electrons from the Earth is believed to neutralize these free radicals, effectively reducing oxidative stress and inflammation. This is similar to taking an over-the-counter medication such as ibuprofen without the potential harmful side effects.[57]

The late Dr. Stephen Sinatra was a pioneer for bringing awareness to the numerous health benefits of grounding, particularly its impact on cardiovascular health. Grounding has been shown to reduce inflammation, improve blood flow, and thin the blood, which helps lower the risk of heart disease and stroke.[58]

Proponents also suggest it can improve metabolic health by neutralizing free radicals and reducing inflammation, a key contributor to chronic diseases like type 2 diabetes and heart disease. Some studies indicate that grounding may lead to improved sleep, reduced pain, and enhanced blood flow, all of which are integral to maintaining metabolic balance.

As of May 2024, the CDC estimates that 119.9 million U.S. adults, or nearly half of the population, have high blood pressure, also known as hypertension. Hypertension is a major risk factor for cardiovascular disease. Studies have found that grounding can lead to notable improvements in blood pressure, suggesting a potential role for grounding in managing and preventing hypertension.[59]

Grounding also promotes a shift from the stress-inducing sympathetic nervous system to the calming parasympathetic nervous system, thereby reducing stress levels and improving sleep quality. Additionally, grounding can enhance heart rate variability (HRV), an important marker of autonomic nervous system balance and overall heart health.[60]

The more you ground, the greater the benefits you'll experience. A good starting point is to ground for 15 to 30 minutes each day to enjoy the wonderful metabolic health advantages I've mentioned.

Walking

Neuroscientist Shane O'Mara has done extensive research on the health benefits of walking and how this simple, everyday activity can profoundly enhance both physical and mental well-being, ultimately promoting longevity. Walking, particularly in natural environments, has been shown to lower blood pressure, improve cardiovascular health, and reduce the risk of chronic diseases such as diabetes and obesity. Regular walking stimulates metabolic processes, aiding in weight management and enhancing the body's ability to regulate blood sugar levels, which are critical components in maintaining metabolic health. O'Mara's findings highlight that even moderate-intensity walking can lead to significant improvements in these areas, contributing to overall better health outcomes.[61]

A recent meta-analysis published by the European Society of Cardiology and the University of Massachusetts Amherst highlights the significant health benefits of walking 5,000 to 7,000 steps per day. This study, which analyzed data from 15 studies involving nearly 50,000 participants, found that walking at least 7,000 steps daily can reduce the risk of all-cause mortality by 50 to 70 percent compared to those who walk fewer steps. This reduction in mortality risk was consistent across different age groups and genders, indicating that increasing daily step count is a universally beneficial strategy for enhancing longevity.[62]

The study also emphasized that even a modest increase in daily steps could lead to substantial health benefits. For example, an additional 1,000 steps per day was associated with a 15 percent reduction in the risk of dying from any cause. Similarly, walking 500 more steps per day correlated with a 7 percent decrease in the risk of cardiovascular disease mortality. These findings suggest that people do not need to reach the often-cited goal of 10,000 steps per day to experience significant health benefits; even moderate increases in physical activity can have profound impacts on health and longevity.[63]

Further supporting these findings, a study from the National Heart, Lung, and Blood Institute (NHLBI) involving more than 2,000 middle-aged adults demonstrated that those who walked at least 7,000 steps per day had a significantly lower risk of death over an 11-year period. The study also found that step intensity did not significantly affect the risk of death, underscoring the importance of total step count over the pace at which the steps are taken. This reinforces the notion that incorporating more steps into daily routines, regardless of speed, can be a simple yet effective way to improve health and extend life expectancy.[64]

Walking after a Meal

Now that we've discussed the health and longevity benefits of walking every day, let's discuss another biohack within walking itself. Walking after a meal can be likened to giving your metabolism a gentle nudge, much like stirring a pot to keep its contents from settling. This simple activity not only aids digestion by encouraging the smooth transit of food through the gastrointestinal tract—thereby reducing bloating and discomfort—but also plays a crucial role in regulating blood sugar levels.

By enhancing glucose uptake by muscles, post-meal walking prevents insulin spikes and the subsequent storage of fat, akin to putting excess energy to immediate use rather than storing it away. This improved blood sugar control is essential for weight management and reduces the risk of developing type 2 diabetes. Additionally, walking increases overall energy expenditure, contributing to a higher calorie burn throughout the day. By incorporating regular post-meal walks, you can effectively boost your metabolic health and support weight loss, turning a simple stroll into a powerful tool for better health.

A study published in the *European Journal of Nutrition* investigated the effects of walking after meals on glucose response with varying carbohydrate content. The study involved healthy young volunteers and found that a 30-minute brisk walk after meals significantly reduced the glucose peak, regardless of the carbohydrate content or macronutrient composition of the meal. The findings suggest that incorporating a brisk walk after eating can improve glycemic control and might be an effective strategy for managing blood sugar levels and enhancing metabolic health.[65]

Meal Pairing

Meal pairing, also known as food sequencing or meal sequencing, involves consuming different types of food in a specific order to optimize metabolic health, particularly blood glucose levels after eating. The concept is based on the idea that the order in which you eat your food can significantly impact how your body processes and responds to different nutrients, especially carbohydrates.

Jessie Inchauspé, a biochemist and founder of the Glucose Goddess movement, has made significant contributions to understanding how meal pairing can optimize metabolic health, facilitate fat loss, and regulate glucose levels after meals. Her research emphasizes the strategic combination of foods to minimize blood sugar spikes, which are critical in managing insulin sensitivity and overall metabolic function. She advocates for the inclusion of fiber, proteins, and healthy fats at the beginning of meals to slow down glucose absorption—this approach helps in maintaining steady blood glucose levels, reducing the risk of metabolic disorders such as diabetes and obesity.

Inchauspé's work also highlights the impact of meal sequencing on fat loss. By preventing large glucose spikes, the body reduces insulin secretion, which is pivotal in fat storage. Lower insulin levels facilitate lipolysis, the breakdown of stored fats into free fatty acids, which the body can then utilize for energy—thus, the deliberate pairing of foods can support weight management and fat-loss efforts. Moreover, her research underscores the importance of avoiding refined carbohydrates and sugars, which contribute to significant glucose fluctuations and subsequent insulin spikes, promoting fat storage.

Inchauspé's research provides practical guidelines for managing post-meal glucose levels. She suggests consuming vinegar-based dressings or a small amount of apple cider vinegar before meals to enhance insulin sensitivity and slow down gastric emptying. Her studies also emphasize the benefit of physical activity post-meal, such as light walking, to facilitate glucose uptake by muscles, thereby reducing blood sugar levels. These simple yet effective strategies are integral to maintaining metabolic health and preventing long-term complications associated with chronic hyperglycemia.[66, 67, 68, 69]

Other studies support Inchauspé's research. A significant one, for instance, found that consuming vegetables and protein before carbohydrates resulted in a substantial reduction in glucose levels after meals. In this study, participants who ate carbohydrates last experienced a 28.6 percent reduction in glucose levels at 30 minutes, a 36.7 percent reduction at 60 minutes, and a 16.8 percent reduction at 120 minutes compared to when they consumed carbohydrates first. Researchers also observed a 73 percent decrease in the incremental area under the curve for glucose, indicating a significant reduction in overall blood glucose exposure over time.[70]

Another study highlighted similar findings, showing that eating carbohydrates last, after protein and vegetables, effectively lowers post-meal glucose spikes. This approach helps to slow down carbohydrate digestion, leading to a more gradual increase in blood glucose levels. This method not only helps manage glucose levels but can also improve insulin sensitivity and overall metabolic health.[71, 72, 73]

What I love about everything I've shared in this book so far is that these tools harness your inner physician (innate intelligence) to go to work for you. Never forget, your body is designed to self-heal. It has the world's greatest physician within every cell, waiting to repair and heal it, as long as you remove the interference.

Now that we've done our job identifying the main interferences and the best tools for harnessing innate intelligence, are you ready to put all this information into action? Then let's get you on your 30-Day Metabolic Freedom Reset!

CHAPTER 12

YOUR 30-DAY METABOLIC FREEDOM RESET

Welcome to your 30-Day Metabolic Freedom Reset, which will help you restore your metabolism by applying the principles you've learned in this book. I designed this reset to give you an easy-to-follow protocol that harnesses the innate intelligence within your cells by using ancient healing practices and the latest cutting-edge science. It has worked on thousands of people across the world—and you're next!

As you may recall, the number one priority for your innate intelligence is survival. Forcing adaptation creates hormone optimization and faster results. Hormone adaptation is the process by which your body adjusts hormone levels in response to external stressors (like exercise, dietary changes, fasting, or temperature changes) to maintain balance and support survival.

You will achieve this during your reset by practicing a new schedule each week to continue forcing hormonal shifts. The 30-day reset will work for someone who has never practiced keto or fasting before or for someone who's been practicing it for years. We're going to utilize metabolic flexing to shift in and out of sugar burning to fat burning. I've also mapped out an advanced version if you've been doing keto and fasting for a while and want a more challenging reset. (Note that it's always best to speak with your doctor and advise them of this new healthy lifestyle you are about to embark upon.)

As a former personal trainer, I understand the proper balance between pushing you outside your comfort zone and pushing you too far, so I designed the reset to push you beyond your comfort zone just enough to ignite healing but not too much where you'll feel miserable and restricted. As Joseph Campbell said, "The cave you fear holds the treasure you seek."

One of the biggest reasons people fail at hitting their goals is because they don't plan for the obstacles that will more than likely show up. It's okay to hit obstacles along the way—success is rarely a straight path. We'll be using hormetic stressors to achieve deep healing and fat burn, and sometimes this can be difficult. Your gut microbiome will shift, your palate will change, and you'll find yourself walking into the kitchen for a snack before becoming aware of what you're doing to stop yourself and stay the course. The truth is, it might suck. Embrace it. Suck, suck, SUCCESS is my philosophy!

Price Pritchett's book *You*[2] emphasizes the concept of quantum leaps in personal achievement.[1] He illustrates this by comparing personal growth to rockets course-correcting their way to the moon, constantly adjusting their trajectory to stay on path and reach their destination. This analogy highlights the importance of continuous, small adjustments and persistence in achieving significant breakthroughs and goals. I always tell my students it's never about the setback, it's about the getback. This book is your resource to course-correct until you achieve success.

Who Is This Reset For?

The 30-Day Metabolic Freedom Reset is for everyone! It's an incredibly effective path to mastering your metabolism for adults of all ages. Although there are numerous health benefits to this reset, here are some of the symptoms and conditions that it helps with the most:

- insulin resistance
- PCOS
- weight-loss resistance
- diabetes
- prediabetes
- cardiovascular conditions
- autoimmune conditions
- brain fog
- memory problems

- mood disorders such as anxiety and depression
- gut dysbiosis (also called leaky gut)
- repairing your gut post antibiotic use
- detoxing from birth control
- hormonal cancers
- menopause symptoms
- low energy
- infertility challenges
- lack of motivation
- accelerated aging
- thyroid conditions
- hair loss

The Benefits of Doing This with a Community

There's a proverb, "If you want to go fast, do it alone. If you want to go far, do it together." The Harvard Study of Adult Development, one of the longest and most comprehensive longitudinal studies ever conducted, reveals the profound benefits of positive relationships on health and happiness.[2] Beginning in 1938, this ongoing research study followed 724 participants from diverse backgrounds over decades. The findings are clear: Those who maintained close, supportive relationships with family, friends, and their community experienced better physical health, greater longevity, and higher levels of happiness and life satisfaction. Strong social ties also provided significant mental health benefits, acting as a buffer against stress and depression, and contributing to overall well-being. This study underscores the critical importance of nurturing positive relationships for a long, happy, and healthy life.

Humans are inherently social creatures who thrive in community settings, which provide us with a sense of identity, purpose, and security. Social connections enhance emotional well-being, foster cooperation, and create a support network that helps us navigate life's challenges. In essence, our need for social interaction and belonging is deeply ingrained, highlighting the fundamental role of community in human life.

There are lots of ways you can build a community around you. Ask a friend or family member to join you in these 30 days, start a book club, or find my online communities over at www.benazadi.com. You're not alone. There are many people out there who seek metabolic freedom. We're all cheering for you.

Becoming Fat-Adapted: The First Step Toward Metabolic Freedom

As we discussed earlier in the book, about 93 percent of U.S. adults are burning sugar instead of fat. The first step toward metabolic freedom is to teach your metabolism to burn fat instead of sugar. This is called fat adaptation, when you are burning stored fat on your body instead of sugar in your bloodstream.

I've guided over 5,000 students through my Keto Kamp Academy online program and helped them burn fat instead of sugar within seven days—without any symptoms! There are four easy ways to achieve this first step: avoid certain foods, follow the 2/2/2 rule, drink a keto cocktail, and avoid snacking between meals. Let's look at each of them in detail.

1. Avoid Certain Foods

There are two primary gatekeepers that block your metabolism from burning stored fat: the hormone insulin and cellular membrane inflammation. Avoiding foods that spike glucose and insulin along with foods that create cellular membrane inflammation will help you shift quickly into fat-burning mode and ensure a successful 30-day reset.

Refined Sugars, Refined Flours, and Most Carbohydrates

The first category of foods to avoid include those that are higher on the glycemic index and will raise your blood glucose after eating them. When you raise blood glucose after eating, the pancreas is signaled to produce insulin to shuttle the excess blood sugar into your cells, and you're burning sugar, not fat. To become fat-adapted and in ketosis within the first seven days of your reset, you need to remove the following foods:

- white bread
- pastries (like donuts, muffins, and cakes)
- sugary breakfast cereals
- cookies and biscuits

- candy and sweets
- sweetened beverages (sodas, energy drinks, and sweetened teas)
- pasta
- pizza
- packaged snack foods (like crackers and chips)
- ice cream and frozen desserts

When it comes to getting your metabolism to burn stored body fat and use ketones as a fuel source, total carbohydrates need to be considered as well. The average American consumes 250 grams of carbohydrates per day; most people need to reduce their total carbohydrates to under 50 total grams per day to achieve fat-burning ketosis.

I don't recommend a sharp reduction in total carbohydrates at the beginning of your reset, because this could result in uncomfortable symptoms such as fatigue, loose stools, and headaches. Instead, a gradual decrease in total carbohydrates works really well. (See page 180 for a list of healthy carbohydrates.) If you're wondering whether fruit is allowed on your plan, the answer is yes, but it depends on the type of fruit and the quantity consumed. The best keto-friendly options include blueberries, raspberries, coconut, avocado, squash, zucchini, and olives.

Here's an example of what this looks like during your first seven days, based on someone who is consuming 250 grams of total carbohydrates per day before starting the reset. Adjust accordingly.

- Day 1: 200 grams of total carbohydrates
- Day 2: 150 grams of total carbohydrates
- Day 3: 100 grams of total carbohydrates
- Day 4: 75 grams of total carbohydrates
- Day 5: 50 grams or less of total carbohydrates

Once you're at 50 grams of total carbohydrates or less for a few days, the metabolic switch to fat-burning ketosis occurs. You can use several free apps to log in your food and calculate your total carbohydrates—a couple of my favorites are Cronometer and MyFitnessPal.

Inflammatory Oils

You also want to avoid inflammatory oils that cause your cells to inflame and make you insulin resistant. These oils make it harder to practice fasting and block you from fat burning, so I highly recommend you throw them out and replace them with the healthier options I will share with you in the next step.

Here's a list of the harmful oils you want to avoid:

- canola oil
- corn oil
- cottonseed oil
- rapeseed oil
- partially hydrogenated oil
- vegetable oil
- sunflower oil
- safflower oil
- soybean oil
- rice bran oil
- grapeseed oil
- refined peanut oil

Chemicals

The third group of foods to remove are the ones filled with chemicals. These are the toxic ingredients I mentioned in Chapter 7 that make you insulin resistant, making it harder to achieve fat adaptation. These ingredients also create cellular inflammation and have been referred to as obesogens and diabetogens.

Common synthetic ingredients to avoid include:

- artificial sweeteners (e.g., aspartame, saccharine, sucralose)
- high-fructose corn syrup (HFCS)
- artificial colors (e.g., Red 40, Yellow 5, Blue 1)
- monosodium glutamate (MSG)
- sodium nitrite and sodium nitrate

- trans fats (partially hydrogenated oils)
- preservatives (e.g., BHA, BHT, TBHQ)
- artificial flavors
- potassium bromate
- propylene glycol

2. Follow the 2/2/2 Rule

This next step should be done in tandem with the previous step. The goal here is to familiarize your metabolism with burning fatty acids instead of sugar. Imagine your metabolism as a seasoned crew navigating a ship that has long relied on sugar as its primary fuel. As you start reducing carbohydrates and eliminating inflammatory foods, the crew becomes anxious, unsure of how to keep the ship sailing without its usual energy source. At this crucial juncture, your body might exhibit signs of distress, akin to a ship adrift without its familiar fuel.

To steady the course and maintain momentum, you need to introduce a new, reliable fuel source: healthy, anti-inflammatory fats. These fats act like a fresh wind in your sails, providing your metabolism with the energy it needs to continue its journey without faltering. By fueling your body with these beneficial fats, you ensure a smooth transition, allowing your metabolic crew to adapt and thrive, navigating the seas of this dietary change with confidence and ease.

The best way to avoid cravings, stabilize your blood sugar, and transition smoothly into fat-burning mode is with the 2/2/2 rule. For the first seven days of your 30-day reset, you will practice the 2/2/2 rule:

- 2 tablespoons of grass-fed butter, grass-fed ghee, beef tallow, or duck fat
- 2 tablespoons of coconut oil or MCT oil
- 2 tablespoons of olive oil or avocado oil

You aren't consuming all these healthy fats in one meal; spread them out throughout your three meals for the day. You'll be using these fats to cook your food in, for salad dressings, dips, and so on. If you feel like this is too much fat to consume in a day, you can change it to the 1/1/1 rule and have one tablespoon of each fat instead of two.

In addition to these fats, you will add the following healthy proteins:

- grass-fed beef
- pork
- lamb
- eggs
- bison
- turkey
- chicken
- charcuterie meats like salami and prosciutto (nitrate free)
- venison (deer)
- wild-caught sardines
- wild-caught salmon

Of course, you want to continue consuming vegetables in your diet for all of their amazing health benefits. Here's a list of the best keto-friendly vegetables:

- broccoli
- Brussels sprouts
- arugula
- asparagus
- cabbage
- mushrooms
- lettuce
- cucumbers
- artichokes
- radishes
- celery

If you're wondering about portion sizes, here's the great news: You don't need to worry about them or count calories, since your body doesn't naturally calculate these things. Instead, focus on eating until you're full. Your body has built-in mechanisms for satiety, and the goal is to feel satisfied, not restricted. Eating until you're full helps prevent cravings between meals and ensures you stay on track.

3. Drink a Keto Cocktail

Carbohydrates are stored in the body with water, so when you reduce your carb intake, your body initially sheds excess water, giving you a quick "lean" appearance. Lowering carbs also reduces insulin release, causing the kidneys to excrete more sodium, which disrupts the balance of essential electrolytes like sodium, potassium, and magnesium. These electrolytes are crucial for hydration, energy production, and overall cell function. As carb intake decreases, electrolyte imbalances can lead to keto flu symptoms like headaches and fatigue.

Ensuring proper hydration and electrolyte intake is essential, which is why I created the Keto Kamp Cocktail. Drink it every morning for at least seven days.

KETO KAMP COCKTAIL

16 ounces spring water

2 tablespoons apple cider vinegar

2 teaspoons cream of tartar (for extra potassium)

1 pinch high-quality salt

Mix all ingredients in a glass and drink.

4. Avoid Snacking Between Meals

Every time you snack, you raise insulin and start the digestive process. This blocks fat burning and steals energy away from your day-to-day activities to deal with digestion. It will be much more difficult to teach your metabolism to burn fat instead of sugar when you're constantly calling insulin.

For the first seven days of your 30-day reset, consume three meals per day, with no snacking in between. For example, your schedule may look like this: breakfast at 8 A.M., lunch at 12 P.M., and dinner at 7 P.M. This allows insulin to drop in between meals and overnight during sleep. If you already practice intermittent fasting, then continue with your preferred fasting schedule for these first seven days.

Metabolic Flex Days

You'll see metabolic flex days as a part of your 30-day reset; I also call them keto flex days. These are days during your plan that intentionally move you out of fat-burning ketosis so that you can burn sugar. This works really well to achieve metabolic flexibility but also allows more flexibility within your plan overall.

Most people are metabolically inflexible because their bodies are "stuck" burning sugar. However, there's also a group on the opposite end who are "stuck" burning fat, which also leads to metabolic inflexibility. The goal is to become efficient at switching between both fuel sources—sugar and fat. Achieving this metabolic flexibility fine-tunes your metabolism and helps prevent or overcome weight-loss stalls.

You can use flex (feast) days when you have social events, such as on the weekend. On these days, you will not be eating keto-friendly foods and practicing fasting. Instead, you will have three meals and bring your total carbohydrates to 150 grams for the day. However, these carbs still need to be healthier versions—no pastries, chips, cookies, pizza, ice cream, and so on from the "foods to avoid" list.

It's important to decrease your total fats as you raise your total carbohydrates, since having higher carbohydrates and higher fat is not healthy for your metabolism. Your total fats should be kept under 50 grams for each metabolic flex day.

Here's a list of healthy carbohydrates to include on your metabolic flex days:

- grapes
- guava
- blackberries
- mango
- coconut
- melons
- cranberries
- papaya
- passion fruit
- plantain
- raspberries
- watermelon
- blueberries
- pineapple
- strawberries
- tangerine
- grapefruit
- pomegranate
- apple
- apricot
- cherries
- figs
- kiwifruit
- lychee
- nectarine
- orange

- peach
- pears
- summer squash
- plums
- bananas
- dates
- arrowroot
- resistant starch powder
- pumpkin
- plantain flour
- butternut squash
- black rice
- sweet potato

- wild rice
- yam
- brown rice
- carrot
- artichokes
- white rice
- zucchini
- cassava
- winter squash
- taro
- green beans
- tapioca flour/starch

Tips for Succeeding at Your Reset

As I mentioned in Chapter 10, your environment will determine your success. So it's a good idea to first do an audit on your home and office environment. Remove foods that tempt you the most—anything that could derail you. One of my favorite foods is popcorn. I could snack on this all day long. But popcorn is high on the glycemic index, so eating this would not be conducive to fat burning. I had to remove popcorn and other trigger foods from my kitchen, because if I knew they were there, I'd end up snacking on them. It wasn't safe to have them in the house. Identify the foods that are not safe for you to have in your house or office, and remove them.

Next, do an audit on your relationship environment. Your friends, family members, and co-workers will either support you or drag you down (remember the crabs in the bucket analogy). I encourage you to do this quick exercise: Grab a blank piece of paper, draw a line vertically through the middle and then one at the top horizontally. On the top left, write the word *drainers*, and on the top right, write the word *chargers*. Then think about the relationships you have. After you think of each person, place them in either the drainer or the charger category.

How do you know if someone is a drainer or a charger? Well, when you have conversations with them, do you feel drained afterward? Are they naysayers? If so, they belong in the drainer category. If you feel charged up and energized after speaking with them, though, and they support your goals, place them in the chargers category. Do this with every person in your life.

After you've completed your audit, it's important to then be sure that you're spending more time with the chargers than with the drainers. I realize this is easier said than done, but you become your environment, and I want you to surround yourself with people who cheer you on through this process, not the crabs who drag you down in the bucket.

Last but not least, create a process that's going to help you change your self-image. Remember, your paradigms are a multitude of habits that guide every move you make. They affect the way you eat, the way you walk, even the way you talk. They govern your communication, your work habits, your successes, and your failures. Your success is highly determined by your paradigm, which creates your self-image. Repetition is how you alter the paradigm to change your self-image to that of a healthy person.

Affirmations are a great way to reinforce the new self-image. Write the following affirmation on an index card or sticky note, and read it each morning and before bed, when the subconscious mind is most impressionable:

"I am so happy and grateful now that I am at my perfect weight. I am looking good, and I am feeling great. The perfect health I seek is now seeking me; I remove any blockages between us."

The more focus and feelings you put into the affirmation, the faster it will work for you. You might want to leave it on your computer screen or refrigerator too!

Take Your Vitamin G Twice Per Day

As you've learned, vitamin G is the most powerful anti-inflammatory supplement there is. But the practice of gratitude is not an intellectual practice—it's an emotional one. Similar to your affirmation, the more senses you bring into this exercise, the faster it will work for you.

Here's your prescription for your 30-day reset: Spend three minutes each morning and evening taking vitamin G. For each minute, focus on a memory or relationship you're truly grateful for—really soak up the vitamin G. After the minute is up, move on to another. Do this for three minutes in the morning and three minutes in the evening before bed. This is when your subconscious mind is most impressionable.

BONUS POINTS: PRACTICE THESE BIOHACKS FOR BETTER RESULTS

The more you put into something, the more you get out of it. If you really want to accelerate your results, then add the following biohacks to your 30-day reset. This is optional and not required for success during your reset:

- Cold therapy (ice bath, plunge, cold shower, cryotherapy): 11 minutes total per week

- Heat therapy (sauna): 60 minutes total per week

- Walking (activity): 10,000 steps per day

- Red light therapy (photobiomodulation): 10 minutes per day

- Grounding/earthing (walking barefoot): 30 minutes per day

The 30-Day Metabolic Freedom Reset

Whenever I start a new goal, I like to see the big picture of what I'm going to be doing. This helps my mind be more receptive to the changes. With that being said, let's get a general overview of what your 30-day reset will look like and then go into the details.

There are three ground rules to remember as you move through this reset: You will avoid inflammatory foods, you will consume an insulin-friendly diet with intentional feast days, and you will experience four different fasting lengths.

Avoid:

- bad oils
- alcohol
- toxic chemical ingredients
- refined flours and sugar

Consume an Insulin-Friendly Diet:

- low-carbohydrate diet
- ketogenic diet
- high-protein ketogenic diet
- metabolic flex (keto flexing)

Type of Fasting:

- intermittent fasting (12 to 16 hours)
- autophagy fasting (18 hours)
- metabolic fasting (20 hours)
- gut-repair fasting (24 hours)

Intentionally choosing foods that support your metabolism can be simple and enjoyable. While we've been conditioned to eat based on taste alone, you'll soon find that your taste buds will begin to crave these delicious, hormone-boosting foods.

To help you succeed with your 30-Day Metabolic Freedom Reset, I've compiled food lists to align with the different food plans/phases that support your microbiome, hormones, liver, and overall metabolism. Here are a few things to keep in mind as you go through these lists:

1. This is a starting point to help you identify foods that can be part of your personalized metabolic freedom lifestyle. If you don't see some of your favorite foods listed, that's okay—the lists are meant to guide you toward metabolic healing.

2. Some foods may appear in multiple categories; these are powerful metabolic superfoods. For example, green leafy vegetables like broccoli, arugula, and Brussels sprouts are excellent for liver health and bile production, so feel free to include them throughout your 30-day plan.

3. Since pesticides can disrupt hormones and negatively impact your metabolism, try to choose organic, non-GMO, and antibiotic-free options whenever possible.

Remember to reference the food lists in Chapter 7 for ketogenic and liver-supporting foods and Chapter 9 for foods that support your metabolism, including probiotic- and prebiotic-rich foods and polyphenol foods. Enjoy experimenting with these delicious, metabolism-supporting foods, and be sure to try the recipes included later in the book that bring these foods to life. Happy fueling on your journey to metabolic freedom!

✦ ✦

Now that we have our three ground rules in place, let's guide you through what your 30-Day Metabolic Freedom Reset will look like. Remember, this reset is designed to remove what's been interfering with your metabolism, so you can balance your hormones to burn fat and feel great. I recommend you follow each day as outlined. Getting fat-adapted is the biggest needle mover to achieve before we get into fasting and other biohacking strategies.

Here's a day-to-day guide to your reset, in which you'll move through these phases: fat adaptation, autophagy, metabolic rebuilding, and metabolic flexing. Enjoy!

1. Fat Adaptation Phase (Days 1 to 6)

The fat adaptation phase is designed to shift your metabolism from burning sugar to burning fat in just one week. Burning fat instead of sugar reduces inflammation in your body and supports your mitochondria, which is crucial for restoring and optimizing your metabolism. I have structured this process to ensure a smooth and effortless transition, so within the first few days, you can expect to experience increased energy levels, improved sleep, and noticeable fat loss.

Food choice throughout the phase: low-carbohydrate diet transition to ketogenic diet. Your first step is to gradually reduce your total carbohydrate intake, which helps lower the fat-storing hormone insulin. By making this change gradually, your metabolism can transition to burning fat for fuel without causing any discomfort. A low-carbohydrate diet typically involves consuming around 75 to 150 grams of total carbohydrates per day. This is an essential first step before moving into a ketogenic diet, which requires reducing your intake to less than 50 grams of carbohydrates per day. Remember to gradually decrease your total carbohydrate intake each day to make the transition smoother.

Low-Carbohydrate Diet

- 75 to 150 grams of total carbohydrates
- 75 grams of protein
- healthy fats as desired

Ketogenic Diet Foods

These foods work well for ketosis days. You will want to put your food focus on these foods during the entire 30-day reset, except for your metabolic flex (keto flex) day, which occurs on days 26 and 30.

Seeds and Nuts

- cashews
- pine nuts
- Brazil nuts
- walnuts
- pumpkin seeds
- sesame seeds
- sunflower seeds
- pistachios
- pecans

Fruits and Vegetables

- arugula
- broccoli
- Brussels sprouts
- cauliflower
- cabbage
- onions

- garlic
- zucchini
- blueberries
- cranberries
- strawberries

Days 1 to 4: intermittent fasting (12 hours) with no snacking between meals. You will eat 3 meals a day—breakfast, lunch, and dinner. For example, if you finish dinner at 8 P.M., you will fast overnight until breakfast at 8 A.M., completing a 12-hour intermittent fast.

Days 5 to 6: intermittent fasting (14 hours). You will continue to eat 3 meals a day, but by either delaying breakfast by 2 hours or eating dinner 2 hours earlier, you can achieve a 14-hour fast. For example, if you finish dinner at 8 P.M., you would fast overnight until breakfast at 10 A.M. Alternatively, you could finish dinner at 6 P.M. and fast until breakfast at 8 A.M., completing a 14-hour intermittent fast. Choose the option that best fits your schedule.

DOES COFFEE OR TEA BREAK A FAST?

This is one of the most common questions I receive on my social media channels. To answer it, we first need to define what it means to "break a fast." My definition of this is when you signal to your body to exit the autophagy state—where it cleans and repairs cells—and shift into the mTOR state, which is anabolic and focused on building up. Blood glucose levels determine whether you're in the fasted state (autophagy) or the fed state (mTOR).

Coffee and tea can have different effects on fasting: For some people, they can stimulate autophagy and enhance fasting benefits; while for others, they may disrupt the fasted state. It's important to note that not all coffee beans are created equal—many coffee beans are loaded with pesticides, heavy metals, and mold, which can spike blood sugar. To avoid this, make sure your coffee is mold- and pesticide-free, and look for beans labeled "organic" or "mold-free" on the packaging. When in doubt, reach out to the company for confirmation. Many coffee shops are proud of their pure coffee and will disclose the sourcing of their beans. Switching to clean coffee beans can often solve the problem of glucose spikes.

The best way to determine if coffee or tea breaks your fast is to test your blood sugar before drinking it and again 45 minutes afterward. If your blood sugar rises by 5 points or more, then it's likely breaking your fast and reducing autophagy benefits.

If your blood sugar stays the same or drops slightly, you're in the clear. Everyone's response is different, so it's important not to guess—test instead.

Consider experimenting with adding fats such as butter, coconut oil, or ghee to your coffee instead of drinking it black, as this can sometimes help stabilize glucose levels. Also, teas are generally safer options when it comes to fasting, as I haven't observed them causing glucose spikes in most people. It's still wise to choose organic teas to ensure purity, though.

2. Autophagy Phase (Days 7 to 13)

As you may remember, autophagy is the process where your body breaks down inflamed cells and damaged mitochondria, repurposing them as fuel. Imagine it like Pac-Man, gobbling up broken cells within your body to use as energy. Autophagy is one of the most effective ways to eliminate unhealthy cells and regenerate healthier ones, which not only boosts your metabolism but also supports longevity.

Food choice throughout the phase: ketogenic diet. At this stage of your reset, we transition into fat-burning ketosis. Ketones are a powerful tool for resetting your metabolism, balancing hormones, sharpening your mind, and burning fat. You'll experience peak mental clarity, increased energy levels and focus, and an overall sense of well-being. To achieve ketosis, it's essential to keep your total carbohydrate intake under 50 grams per day, focusing on non-starchy vegetables and the low-glycemic fruits mentioned earlier in this chapter.

Ketogenic Diet

- 50 grams of total carbohydrates or less
- 75 grams of protein
- healthy fats as desired

Days 7 to 13: autophagy fasting (18 hours). Now it's time to experiment with meal-skipping. Since you're fat-adapted and running on ketones, this experience should be enjoyable. You'll be following an 18/6 intermittent fasting schedule to promote autophagy. This means you'll spend 18 hours in a fasted state and have a 6-hour eating window, during which you'll consume two keto-friendly meals. For example, you might start your eating window at 12 P.M. with your first meal, and finish your last meal by 6 P.M., then fast from 6 P.M. until 12 P.M. the next day (18 hours). Alternatively, you could have breakfast at 8 A.M., lunch at 2 P.M., and then fast from 2 P.M. until 8 A.M. the next day (18 hours). Both methods are effective, so choose the fasting schedule that best fits your lifestyle.

3. Metabolic Rebuilding Phase (Days 14 to 20)

The metabolic rebuilding phase is where we fine-tune your metabolism. We'll do this by extending your fasting window slightly to enhance autophagy and further lower insulin levels. Additionally, we'll shift to a protein-focused ketogenic diet, emphasizing high-quality amino acids. The increased protein intake will help sustain you during longer fasts and make your metabolism more efficient by balancing key hormones.

Food choice throughout the phase: high-protein ketogenic diet. A typical keto diet is usually high in fat, with moderate protein and very low carbohydrates. However, during the metabolic rebuilding phase, we increase protein intake to leverage the benefits of amino acids for hormone health and metabolic repair. Aim to consume at least 40 grams of protein with each meal. There's no need to focus on additional fat at this stage, as your body will use stored fat for fuel. Simply consume the fat that naturally comes with your protein sources. Keep total carbohydrates under 50 grams per day to stay in ketosis.

High-Protein Ketogenic Diet

- 50 grams of total carbohydrates or less
- 1 gram of protein per pound of ideal body weight
- healthy fats that come naturally with protein

High-Protein Keto Foods

Integrating these proteins into your diet all month long is a good idea, especially during your metabolic rebuilding phase (days 14 to 20).

- Eggs
- Turkey
- Chicken
- Cottage cheese
- Shellfish
- Red meat, such as lamb and beef
- Pork
- Chia seeds
- Tofu
- Quinoa

Days 14 to 20: metabolic fasting (20 hours). You will consume two high-protein keto meals within a 4-hour eating window. For example, you might eat between 12 P.M. and 4 P.M., then fast from 4 P.M. until 12 P.M. the next day. Alternatively, you could eat between 8 A.M. and 12 P.M., followed by a fast from 12 P.M. until 8 A.M. the next day. Choose the schedule that fits your lifestyle best.

4. Metabolic Flexing Phase (Days 26 and 30)

The metabolic flexing phase is designed to maintain your metabolic flexibility while making it easier to navigate social events. The goal is to switch between burning sugar and fat for energy, and this phase intentionally alternates between the two. By briefly returning to sugar burning before switching back to fat burning, you can prevent and even break through plateaus.

Food choice through the phase: ketosis and metabolic flex days (keto flexing). During your metabolic flex days (keto flexing), you will have a 12-hour eating window and consume three meals within this window. The meals will be higher in carbohydrates to ensure switching back to sugar burning for the day. Aim to consume

150 grams of total carbohydrates on these metabolic flex days, coming from healthy carbohydrates.

Metabolic Flex Days (Keto Flexing)

- 100 to 150 grams of total carbohydrates
- 1 gram of protein per pound of ideal body weight
- less than 50 total grams of healthy fats

Metabolic Flex Day Foods

These foods are perfect for your metabolic flex (keto flex) days. The vegetables will balance your hormones and provide healthy sources of carbohydrates to flex out of ketosis. You want to consume these foods during your metabolic flex, which are days 26 and 30 of your plan.

Root Vegetables

- white potatoes
- red potatoes
- sweet potatoes
- turnips
- pumpkin
- butternut squash
- acorn squash
- honeynut squash
- spaghetti squash
- yams
- yucca (cassava)

Tropical Fruits

- mango
- pineapple
- papaya
- guava
- passion fruit
- lychee
- dragon fruit (pitaya)
- coconut
- banana

Citrus Fruits

- orange
- lemon
- lime
- grapefruit
- tangerine
- mandarin
- clementine

Days 21 to 25: metabolic fasting (20 hours) and high-protein ketogenic diet. You will consume 2 high-protein keto meals within a 4-hour eating window.

Day 26: metabolic flex day/keto flexing (intermittent fasting 12 hours). You will consume breakfast, lunch, and dinner for a total of 3 meals.

Days 27 to 29: metabolic fasting (20 hours) and high-protein ketogenic diet. You will consume 2 high-protein keto meals within a 4-hour eating window.

Day 30: metabolic flex day/keto flexing (intermittent fasting 12 hours). You will consume breakfast, lunch, and dinner for a total of 3 meals.

Advanced Fasting Reset

If you're already fat-adapted by following a ketogenic diet with intermittent fasting, follow this advanced version of the 30-day reset. Longer fasts and more variation in your fasting schedule will allow just enough hormetic stress to naturally force your body to adapt to make that jump to the next level of health.

1. Fat Adaptation Phase Advanced—Deep Ketosis

Days 1 to 4: autophagy fasting (18 hours)
Days 5 to 6: gut-repair fasting (24 hours)

2. Autophagy Phase Advanced—Fat-Focused Foods

Days 7 to 13: Alternate between autophagy fasting (18 hours) and metabolic fasting (20 hours)

3. Metabolic Rebuilding Phase Advanced—Protein-Focused Foods

Days 14 to 20: Alternate between metabolic fasting (20 hours) and gut-repair fasting (24 hours)

4. Metabolic Flexing Phase Advanced—Keto Flexing

Days 21 to 25: metabolic fasting (20 hours)
Day 26: metabolic flex day/keto flexing (12-hour intermittent fasting)
Days 27 to 30 gut-repair fasting (24 hours)

Hacks to Keep You on Track

There are a lot of moving parts with this reset that extend beyond tracking total weight loss—in fact, the weight you lose will be a side effect of restoring your metabolic health. There are a few tools that can help you track what I call non-scale victories (NSVs). NSVs include but are not limited to the following:

- how your clothes fit
- your energy levels
- your level of confidence
- your sleep quality
- your fitness and mobility
- your digestive health
- your skin complexion
- your body fat percentage

Now, we've all heard the saying "Patience is a virtue," but I have to admit, patience isn't my strong suit—I'm always on the lookout for shortcuts to success. I love sharing these shortcuts, or "hacks," with my community, helping them achieve double the results in half the time.

While these hacks can accelerate the healing process and help you avoid plateaus, it's important to remember that healing isn't always about speed. The time it takes to heal can vary, as someone with more challenges may need more time compared to someone with fewer obstacles affecting their metabolism. The ancient healing principles I've shared with you are effective for everyone, even those dealing with chronic conditions, but healing takes time. Trust the process. It's not about perfection; it's about progress. Your only competition is who you were yesterday, and the goal is to be better than you were the day before.

Think of it like learning to play the piano: It takes practice to hit the keys perfectly. Each day you practice, you get closer to your goal, as long as you stay consistent. Apply these health tips in the same way: If you set a goal to fast for 20 hours but only manage 16, that's still a win. There's no such thing as a failed fast—you've made progress, and that's what matters. The more you apply these principles, the more you'll remove the obstacles in your way, placing your body in the best possible state for healing.

On my Ben Azadi YouTube channel, I often say that knowledge is potential power. It's the consistent application of that knowledge that transforms it into true power. So the more you practice these principles, the easier they will become.

Let's dive into the shortcuts that can help you achieve faster results. You'll learn the most common hacks my community uses to excel in creating metabolic freedom, along with answers to the most frequently asked questions I've received over the years. Read through them and remember to return to this section whenever you encounter an obstacle or need a bit of inspiration. Here we go!

Measuring Blood Sugar and Ketones

One of my favorite tools for tracking metabolic progress is monitoring blood sugar and ketones. If you know someone who is diabetic, you've probably seen them do this before. With modern technology, now you can track these numbers too.

For monitoring glucose, there are two great options available to you: finger prick testing where you prick your finger and place a drop of blood on a small stick that measures your blood sugar and ketones or a continuous glucose monitor (CGM), which I mentioned in Chapter 11. A CGM will give you a continual reading of what your blood sugar is doing without having to prick your finger, but the drawback is that it won't give you a ketone reading.

When it comes to measuring ketones, there are three methods, each corresponding to the three types of ketones: beta-hydroxybutyrate (BHB), acetone, and acetoacetate. Blood tests measure BHB, breathalyzers assess acetone, and urine strips test for acetoacetate. It's advisable to avoid urine strips, as they can be inaccurate, particularly when your body becomes efficient at using ketones, potentially leading to a false negative. Breathalyzers are a good alternative since they don't require finger pricking, though they won't provide a glucose reading. The most reliable method is blood testing for BHB, which is considered the gold standard.

If you choose to track these metrics, there are three key times to test. The first measurement to track is your morning reading. When you wake up in the morning, having fasted overnight, take a blood glucose and ketone reading right away—before your coffee or breakfast. An optimal blood sugar reading is in the range of 70 to 90 mg/dL (milligrams per deciliter). For most of you, with the exception of those doing the Advanced Metabolic Freedom Reset, your ketones will be low and nonexistent during the first few days of your reset. By the end of your fat adaptation phase, day 6, you should be fat-adapted and see ketones at 0.5 mmol/L (millimoles per liter) or higher; this means you're officially burning fat instead of sugar. In other words, you're in ketosis.

The second reading to pay attention to once you begin intermittent fasting 18 hours or more is right before you eat your first meal of the day. Ideally, your blood sugar should be lower before your first meal compared to the morning reading, and your ketones should be higher. This is a good sign that your body is using stored fat for energy and using it efficiently. Ketones are simply a by-product of fat burning.

Let's look at a real-life example. Let's say you wake up at 6 A.M., and your readings are 105 mg/dL for your blood sugar and 0.3 mmol/L for ketones. Right before you have your first meal of the day a few hours later, you want to see your blood sugar fall below 105 mg/dL and your ketones rise above 0.3 mmol/L. If you see this trend, your body is making a great shift into fat adaptation. Celebrate this win because what you appreciate, appreciates. Over a short period of time, you will continue to see improved numbers.

The third reading you can take is after eating, which will help you see how efficient you were at metabolizing your foods. Testing your blood sugar and ketones two hours after you eat will give you some great insights. For example, if you break your fast at noon, and your blood sugar was at 85 mg/dL and ketones were 0.6 mmol/L, two hours after eating your blood sugar should be back down close to 85 mg/dL and ketones should be around the same level of 0.6 mmol/L or higher. If you see this trend, congrats—you're insulin sensitive, and your metabolism is functioning the way it was designed. If it's not close to the original numbers, don't worry. As you progress through your reset, you'll train your metabolism to become more efficient and insulin sensitive in a short amount of time.

Knowing these numbers serves many benefits, and it can be extremely motivating to see them trend in the right direction. Tracking these numbers and paying attention to how you feel through the 30-day reset is arguably more important than the total number on the weight scale. Remember, your extra weight is a symptom of metabolic dysfunction—as you become healthy, the weight comes off (and stays off) as a side effect.

If you don't want to (or can't) test your blood throughout the day, there are other positive ways to tell if you're in ketosis. First, you'll likely notice reduced hunger, as ketones help regulate appetite naturally. You might also feel an increase in mental clarity and experience a steady, lasting energy throughout the day, as your brain and body efficiently utilize ketones for fuel. Many people report weight loss and feel lighter and less bloated as the body sheds water weight in the early stages. Enhanced focus, improved mood stability, and an overall sense of mental sharpness are other positive signs that ketosis is working for you.

Tips for Decreasing Your Blood Sugar

It's common to struggle to lower your blood sugar levels as you begin the metabolic freedom lifestyle. This is because you're still training your body to burn fat instead of sugar (fat adaptation). But if you're doing all the right things and still have elevated blood sugar levels and can't achieve ketosis, these are the hacks I recommend. You might have to try each one before you find the perfect fit for you.

Hack #1: Lower Your Carbohydrates

In general, most people can achieve ketosis by dropping their total carbohydrates to 50 grams per day. Others may need to be more restrictive, usually those who have been sugar burners for a long time. The solution is to drop your carbohydrates to below 20 grams per day. This isn't a long-term solution, but it can force your body to choose fat.

Keep an eye out for "carbohydrate creep"! This refers to the gradual, often unintentional, increase in carbohydrate intake that can occur when following a ketogenic diet. The keto diet is a low-carb, high-fat eating plan designed to keep your body in a state of ketosis, where it burns fat for fuel instead of carbohydrates. To maintain ketosis, most people aim to keep their daily carb intake very low, typically between 20 to 50 grams of net carbs per day. However, over time, small amounts of carbs can start to sneak back into your diet, leading to carbohydrate creep.

This phenomenon can happen for several reasons. First, portion control of carbs can become more relaxed as you become accustomed to the diet. What starts as strict portion management can gradually shift to more generous servings, and even small increases in carb-rich foods can add up over time. Hidden carbs are another culprit. Many foods, especially processed or packaged ones, contain carbohydrates that aren't immediately obvious. Ingredients like sauces, dressings, or even certain vegetables (potatoes, sweet potatoes, corn, parsnips, beets) can have more carbs than you may realize, contributing to your overall intake. Some keto-friendly foods may even have higher carb counts than expected. Without careful tracking, these can all add up, making it easy to unintentionally increase your carbohydrate intake. The problem with carbohydrate creep is that it can kick you out of ketosis, potentially stalling your weight loss or even causing weight gain. It can also lead to fluctuations in energy levels and cravings, making it harder to stick to the diet.

To prevent carbohydrate creep, it's essential to regularly track your intake, especially when trying new foods. Reading labels carefully is crucial to spot hidden carbs in packaged foods. Focusing on whole, unprocessed foods where carb counts are easier to manage can also help. I recommend using free food journaling apps that calculate your carbohydrates for you.

Hack #2: Prioritize Quality Sleep

When your sleep quality is compromised, it can trigger a cascade of physiological responses that significantly impact your metabolic health. One of the primary consequences of poor sleep is the elevation of stress hormones in your body, particularly cortisol. Elevated cortisol levels are a signal to your body that it's under stress, which can hinder your ability to enter or maintain ketosis.

In addition, elevated cortisol can lead to higher blood sugar levels, which, in turn, can increase insulin production and make it more difficult for your body to burn fat. The result is a metabolic environment that favors fat storage rather than fat burning, effectively sabotaging your efforts to achieve and maintain ketosis.

Poor sleep also affects the production of ghrelin, the hormone responsible for stimulating hunger. When you're sleep-deprived, your body produces more ghrelin, leading to increased appetite and cravings, particularly for high-carb and sugary foods. This hormonal imbalance not only makes it harder to adhere to a ketogenic diet but can lead to overeating, weight gain, and further disruption of your metabolic processes as well.

In essence, sleep is a critical component of metabolic health. Without adequate sleep, your body is more likely to be in a state of stress, with elevated cortisol, glucose, and ghrelin levels. This hampers your ability to achieve ketosis and undermines your overall metabolic efficiency, making it more challenging to reach your health goals. Prioritizing good sleep is therefore not just about feeling rested; it's about creating the optimal conditions for your body to function at its best, metabolize efficiently, and maintain a state of ketosis.

Hack #3: Avoid ALL Processed Foods

Processed foods can severely disrupt your metabolism by leading to insulin resistance. Removing them from your diet can significantly enhance your ability to burn fat and produce ketones. Bad oils, refined sugars, flours, and harmful chemicals keep your body stuck in sugar-burning mode.

I've seen many people follow ketosis and fasting protocols perfectly, yet still consume processed foods during their eating window, which keeps them from entering ketosis. Remember, the Standard American Diet is a major contributor to insulin resistance and inflammation, preventing the metabolism from effectively burning fat.

The three main offenders we've discussed—bad oils, sugar, and chemicals—are critical to avoid. Be sure to read food labels carefully.

Hack #4: Protect Your Liver

The liver, the hardest-working organ in the human body, is what senses the decrease in blood sugar and makes the switch over to ketosis. Yet I have found after taking over 5,000 people through a ketogenic protocol that the number one reason they struggle to shift into ketosis is a sluggish, backed-up liver. If your liver is congested and not performing at its best, you may struggle to make the switch yourself. Be sure to minimize habits that impair the liver, like drug and alcohol use.

A healthy liver is key for success when it comes to metabolic freedom. Eating the bitter-rich foods I outlined for you on page 92 will help, and here are my favorite liver hacks:

- **Coffee enemas:** A coffee enema involves introducing brewed coffee into the colon, which stimulates liver detoxification and cleanses the colon. The caffeine is absorbed through the colon, potentially boosting bile production and aiding toxin removal. Kits available online typically include an enema bag, tubing, and organic coffee, making it easy for users to perform the procedure at home.

- **Castor oil packs:** A castor oil pack involves applying a cloth soaked in castor oil to the skin, typically over the liver area, to promote detoxification, reduce inflammation, and support digestion. The oil is absorbed through the skin, and it's believed to enhance lymphatic circulation and improve liver function. Kits available online usually include organic castor oil, a reusable flannel cloth, and a wrap or heating pad to keep the pack in place, making it easy to use at home.

- **Infrared saunas:** Infrared saunas use infrared light to generate heat, penetrating deeper into the body than traditional saunas. This deep heat promotes sweating, which can aid in the detoxification process by helping to eliminate toxins through the skin, reducing the burden on the liver. Regular use of infrared saunas is believed to support liver health by enhancing circulation and boosting the body's natural detox pathways. Infrared sauna units and portable versions are available online, allowing for convenient use at home.

- **Essential oils:** Certain essential oils—like rosemary, lemon, and geranium—are believed to support liver health by promoting detoxification and reducing inflammation. These oils can be applied topically (diluted with a carrier oil) over the liver area or diffused for inhalation. Kits specifically designed for liver support are available online, often including a selection of oils known for their detoxifying properties.

Hack #5: Reduce Your Toxic Load

Removing toxins from your environment and diet is a powerful way to support liver health. The organ's primary role is to filter and eliminate toxins from the body, so reducing exposure to harmful substances can ease its workload and enhance its function. This includes avoiding processed foods, limiting alcohol, choosing organic produce, and using natural cleaning and personal care products. The big toxins are the heavy metals found in large fish and silver amalgam fillings: these destroy mitochondrial health and severely impact the liver's function.

Hack #6: Support Your Adrenal Glands

Supporting the adrenal glands is key for blood sugar regulation and achieving ketosis, as these glands produce hormones like cortisol that influence blood sugar levels. Chronic stress can overwork the adrenals, leading to imbalances that make it harder to stabilize blood sugar and enter ketosis. To support adrenal health, focus on stress management with practices like meditation and grounding, adequate sleep, and a diet rich in nutrients like magnesium and B vitamins. Remember to get your daily dose of vitamin G (gratitude), as this automatically lowers cortisol levels.

Handling Hunger When Fasting

Many people considering fasting worry that they'll feel hungry during their fasting window. In fact, this is one of the most common concerns raised on my YouTube channel. The good news is that once you've completed the fat adaptation phase (days 1 to 6), fasting becomes much easier. Without fat adaptation, hunger can indeed be a challenge, as your body and brain have been relying on glucose for energy for years.

If you start fasting as a sugar burner, your brain's glucose levels will begin to drop, causing it to panic and send intense hunger signals, urging you to seek food, especially quick sources of energy like processed carbs. This hunger is real and can seriously disrupt your fasting efforts.

However, when you're fat-adapted, as glucose levels drop, your brain seamlessly switches to using circulating ketones for energy. These ketones signal to your brain, "You're fine; use me as an energy source." Ketones have been shown to curb cravings and keep hunger at bay.

Now, if you're fat-adapted and still experience hunger during a fast, there are strategies you can use. First, it's important to understand that the hunger hormone ghrelin, like other hormones, is pulsatile—it spikes and then subsides like a wave.

If you think of hunger as a wave, you can be sure that it will eventually pass. To make these hunger waves smaller and less frequent, keep yourself busy. Many people snack out of boredom, seeking a dopamine hit from food. Snacking often becomes an emotional event. Staying occupied with a task can help you ride out the hunger wave, and by the time you're done, the wave may have already diminished. For me, I find that a 10- to 15-minute walk works wonders for this.

Another potential cause of hunger during fasting is a loss of key minerals, such as magnesium, potassium, and sodium. This can trigger hunger signals because your body associates such deficiencies with a need for more nutrients. Sodium in particular plays a crucial role in fluid balance and nerve function, so when levels drop, the body might mistakenly signal hunger to restore balance. To prevent this, I recommend taking electrolytes during your fast. My personal favorites are Beam Minerals, Redmond, and Keto Chow.

If you've tried the first two tips and you're still feeling hungry, there's another great option: consuming healthy fats during your fasting window. Healthy fats can calm hunger and provide satiety without spiking glucose or significantly raising insulin levels, so you remain in a fasted state. A tablespoon of coconut oil, grass-fed butter, or olive oil can be a great fasting snack. You can take them raw by the spoonful or add them to your coffee or tea during your fast.

Dealing with Detox Symptoms

When making dietary changes for the first time, it's common to experience symptoms, similar to how you might feel muscle soreness after working out for the first time in years. The most common symptoms when transitioning to fat adaptation and ketosis can include rashes, muscle aches, headaches, constipation, and fatigue. These symptoms, known as the "keto flu," are often due to a loss of electrolytes. To prevent this, drink the keto cocktail on page 179 and maintain your electrolyte levels by incorporating them into your daily routine. The gradual decrease in carbohydrates during the fat adaptation phase (days 1 to 6) helps your body adjust to the changes, significantly reducing or even preventing symptoms altogether.

If you followed the steps as outlined and are still experiencing detox symptoms, I recommend three things. First, remember that this is your journey, and you should go at your own pace. While I provide the exact steps to achieve metabolic freedom within 30 days, it's perfectly okay if you need more time. If you choose to spend additional time in any of the four phases, I fully support your decision.

Second, make sure that your downstream detox pathways are open, so toxins can effectively move through your body. These pathways include your liver, kidneys, gut, lymphatic system, and skin. As you become an efficient fat burner, your metabolism will tap into stored body fat for energy. For some people who have stored a significant amount of toxins in their fat, this can trigger detox symptoms. When your body detoxifies, it must push these toxins through one of the pathways mentioned.

There are several ways to open your detox pathways, and here are my favorite methods:

- **Lymph massage:** Lymphatic massage is a gentle technique designed to stimulate the flow of lymph fluid, which is essential for detoxifying the body. By encouraging lymphatic circulation, this massage helps remove toxins, waste products, and excess fluids from tissues, promoting overall detoxification and reducing inflammation. Additionally, it supports immune function by enhancing the body's ability to filter and eliminate harmful substances.

- **Dry brushing:** Dry brushing is a simple yet effective technique that promotes detoxification by stimulating the lymphatic system and enhancing circulation. By brushing the skin in a specific pattern, it encourages the movement of lymph fluid, aiding in the removal of toxins and waste products from the body. This practice also exfoliates the skin, removing dead cells and unclogging pores, which further supports the body's natural detox processes. Regular dry brushing can leave the skin smoother, improve circulation, and contribute to overall health by helping to clear out harmful substances.

- **Sweating:** Sweating is a natural and powerful way for the body to detoxify and maintain overall health. Through the process of perspiration, the body releases toxins, including heavy metals and chemicals, which are flushed out through the skin. Sweating also helps regulate body temperature and can support cardiovascular health by improving circulation. Engaging in activities that induce sweating, such as exercise or sauna sessions, not only promotes detoxification but also enhances skin health by unclogging pores and removing impurities. Regular sweating is an essential part of the body's natural detox process, contributing to a cleaner, healthier system.

- **Epsom salt bath:** An Epsom salt bath is a soothing and effective method for promoting detoxification and relaxation. The magnesium sulfate in Epsom salts is easily absorbed through the skin, helping to draw out toxins, reduce inflammation, and relieve muscle tension. This type of bath enhances the body's detoxification process by stimulating the lymphatic system and encouraging the elimination of waste products. Additionally, the magnesium in Epsom salts supports overall health by reducing stress, improving sleep quality, and aiding in muscle recovery.

The third and final tip is to incorporate strong binders, such as zeolite or activated charcoal, into your detox regimen. Zeolite, with its unique crystalline structure and negative charge, helps draw out positively charged toxins like heavy metals and environmental pollutants from your cells, supporting systemic detoxification. Activated charcoal, on the other hand, remains in the gut, acting like a sponge to trap and hold toxins, preventing their reabsorption into the bloodstream. Together, these binders work synergistically to facilitate toxin removal from your body, ensuring they are safely and effectively excreted. My top choice for zeolite is CytoDetox by 180° Solutions, and for binders, I recommend Gut CLR™ from Cellular Solutions.

As you progress through your 30-day reset, your cells will continuously regenerate, becoming healthier. During this process, unhealthy cells may release toxins as they undergo autophagy, and binders play a crucial role in capturing these toxins and ensuring that they are safely eliminated from your body.

As you get ready to embark upon your 30-day reset, there's one thing I want you to remember: It's your race, your pace. Don't beat yourself up for making a mistake or slipping one day. Sometimes you win, sometimes you learn. This is just your paradigm trying to course-correct, and you may want to focus on those affirmations for help. If you feel like sticking with a certain phase longer than the way it's laid out for you, that's totally fine. This should be fun!

Pay close attention to the many positive changes that will happen during this reset. If you get stuck or feel discouraged, lean in to your community and find those chargers in your life to root for you. Go into this reset believing you can do this and that you will achieve great results. If you lack this belief because of your old conditioning (paradigms), then borrow my belief in you until you develop it for yourself. I'm here on the sidelines rooting for you!

RECIPES

BREAKFAST

BROCCOLI FRITTATA

Makes 2 servings

1 cup broccoli florets
2 tablespoons butter
10 large eggs
2 tablespoons finely chopped parsley
½ teaspoon sea salt
¼ teaspoon ground black pepper

Preheat the oven to 375° F.

Blanch the broccoli in a pot of boiling salted water until it's bright green and tender-crisp, about 6 to 8 minutes. Drain the broccoli and set it aside.

Heat the butter in an oven-safe skillet set over medium heat. Whisk the eggs with the parsley, salt, and pepper until combined. Add the broccoli to the skillet in an even layer and pour the egg mixture over the top.

Place a fitted lid on the skillet, place it in the oven, and cook the frittata until the eggs are set, about 20 to 25 minutes.

Slice the frittata into 8 wedges and serve immediately.

Tip: If you don't have a lid for your skillet, place a sheet of aluminum foil on top of the skillet and pinch the edges to seal in the steam.

Nutritional Information
Per serving
Total Fat: 35.5 grams
Protein: 33 grams
Total Carbohydrates: 4.5 grams

TACO OMELETTE

Makes 2 servings

½ pound ground beef

½ teaspoon chili powder

½ teaspoon ground cumin

½ teaspoon dried oregano

½ teaspoon sea salt

¼ teaspoon garlic powder

¼ teaspoon onion powder

¼ teaspoon ground black pepper

2 teaspoons butter, divided

6 large eggs, divided

½ avocado, sliced and divided

2 tablespoons chopped cilantro

2 lime wedges

Heat a skillet set over medium heat. Add the ground beef, chili powder, cumin, oregano, salt, garlic powder, onion powder, and black pepper. Cook, breaking the meat apart with a spatula, until browned and cooked through, about 8 to 10 minutes.

Heat 1 teaspoon of the butter in a large nonstick skillet over medium heat. Whisk the eggs until the mixture is smooth. Pour half of the egg mixture into the skillet and cook it until it's almost set, about 3 to 5 minutes, reducing the heat if needed to prevent overbrowning.

Place half the ground beef mixture on one half of the omelette. Arrange half the avocado slices on top of the ground beef and fold the other half of the omelette over the top. Allow the omelette to cook for another 2 to 3 minutes.

Repeat the process with the remaining ingredients to make a second omelette.

Serve the omelettes with some cilantro sprinkled on top and the lime wedges on the side to squeeze over the top.

Nutritional Information
Per serving
Total Fat: 35.5 grams
Protein: 43.5 grams
Total Carbohydrates: 6.5 grams

TURKEY SAUSAGE MEATBALLS AND EGGS

Makes 2 servings

3 tablespoons butter, divided
10 ounces ground turkey
½ teaspoon Italian seasoning
½ teaspoon fennel seeds
½ teaspoon paprika
½ teaspoon onion powder
½ teaspoon sea salt
¼ teaspoon ground nutmeg
¼ teaspoon ground black pepper
1 garlic clove, minced
4 large eggs

Preheat the oven to 350° F. Line a small baking sheet with parchment paper.

Melt 2 tablespoons of the butter. In a bowl, gently knead the ground turkey with the melted butter, Italian seasoning, fennel seeds, paprika, onion powder, salt, nutmeg, pepper, and garlic until combined. Divide and shape the mixture into 10 meatballs, using a tablespoon to measure them, and place them on the prepared baking sheet.

Bake the meatballs, turning them once, until they are cooked through, about 25 to 30 minutes.

When the meatballs are almost cooked through, heat the remaining butter in a large skillet over medium heat. Add the eggs and cook them sunny-side up, about 3 to 4 minutes. Alternatively, you can cook the eggs in any other style you prefer.

Serve the meatballs with the eggs.

Tip: Wet your hands to make rolling the meatballs easier.

Nutritional Information
Per serving
Total Fat: 35.5 grams
Protein: 43.5 grams
Total Carbohydrates: 6.5 grams

SCRAMBLED EGG TACO BOWLS

Makes 2 servings

1 cup shredded pecorino romano cheese

1 tablespoon butter

8 large eggs

¼ cup chopped cilantro

½ teaspoon sugar-free taco seasoning

Preheat the oven to 400° F. Line a large baking sheet with parchment paper.

Arrange the cheese into two roughly 6-inch circles on the baking sheet, ensuring that it is in a thin even layer. Bake for 6 to 8 minutes, or until cheese is melted and starting to turn golden around the edges. Remove the baking sheet from the oven and immediately place each cheese round on top of the base of a small bowl and gently form each round of cheese around the bowls; allow them to cool.

Heat the butter in a nonstick skillet over medium heat.

Beat the eggs until the mixture is smooth. Pour them into the skillet and scramble until cooked through, about 3 to 5 minutes.

Remove the cheese "taco bowls" from the molds and place them on a plate with the hollow sides facing up. Divide the scrambled eggs between the taco bowls and garnish them with cilantro and a dusting of taco seasoning.

Tip: Make sure the bowls you use to create the taco bowls have a small enough bottom so that the cheese can drape over it and create a bowl deep enough to hold all the eggs. However, don't worry if you can't fit all the eggs in the taco bowls. You can simply enjoy them on the side.

Nutritional Information
Per serving
Total Fat: 37.5 grams
Protein: 33.5 grams
Total Carbohydrates: 2.5 grams

EGG AND PROSCIUTTO CUPS

Makes 2 servings

2 tablespoons melted butter
8 slices prosciutto
8 large eggs
Sea salt and ground black pepper, to taste
¼ cup chopped chives

Preheat the oven to 350° F.

Grease eight cups of a muffin tin with the butter.

Line each muffin cup with 1 slice of prosciutto, so that it covers the bottom and sides. Crack an egg into each cup and season it with salt and pepper to taste.

Bake the eggs until they're set, about 20 minutes.

Divide the cups between two plates, garnish with the chives, and serve immediately.

Nutritional Information
Per serving
Total Fat: 33.5 grams
Protein: 35 grams
Total Carbohydrates: 2 grams

HIGH-PROTEIN BREAKFAST PIZZA

Makes 2 servings

3 tablespoons butter, divided

1 cup sliced mushrooms

¼ teaspoon sea salt

¼ teaspoon ground black pepper

12 large egg whites

1 cup grated pecorino romano cheese

1 teaspoon dried oregano

4 ounces sliced sugar-free pepperoni

Preheat the oven to 350° F. Line two large baking sheets with parchment paper and lightly grease the paper with 1 tablespoon of the butter.

Heat the remaining butter in a skillet over medium heat. Add the mushrooms, salt, and pepper, and cook until golden, about 8 to 10 minutes.

In a large bowl, beat the egg whites until stiff peaks are formed. Place half of the egg whites on each baking sheet and spread them out into two roughly 12-inch circles. Bake until the "pizza crusts" are set, about 20 minutes.

Top the egg white crusts with the cheese, oregano, mushrooms, and pepperoni. Bake until the cheese is melted and the pepperoni is starting to crisp up, about 15 minutes.

Cut the pizzas in slices, divide them between two plates, and serve immediately.

Nutritional Information
Per serving
Total Fat: 34.5 grams
Protein: 41.5 grams
Total Carbohydrates: 3 grams

BREAKFAST CASSEROLE

Makes 2 servings

8 ounces ground beef

½ cup sliced mushrooms

¼ cup chopped red, orange, or yellow bell pepper

½ teaspoon dried oregano

½ teaspoon sea salt

¼ teaspoon ground black pepper

10 large eggs

¼ cup heavy cream

Preheat the oven to 350° F.

Cook the ground beef, mushrooms, bell pepper, oregano, salt, and pepper in a skillet over medium heat until the ground beef and mushrooms are golden and the bell pepper is tender, about 10 minutes. Place the meat mixture in a 9 x 9-inch baking dish.

Whisk the eggs with the heavy cream. Pour the eggs over the meat mixture in the baking dish.

Bake the casserole until it sets and is cooked through, about 35 to 40 minutes.

Cut the casserole into 4 squares, divide it between two plates, and serve immediately.

Nutritional Information
Per serving
Total Fat: 46 grams
Protein: 55 grams
Total Carbohydrates: 4.5 grams

KETO CRUSTLESS QUICHE

Makes 2 servings

1 tablespoon butter

1 cup finely chopped broccoli

1 cup chopped red bell pepper

½ cup chopped onion

6 large eggs

1 cup heavy cream

4 ounces shredded sheep's milk cheddar

¼ teaspoon sea salt

¼ teaspoon ground black pepper

Preheat the oven to 350° F.

Heat the butter in a skillet over medium heat. Add the broccoli, red bell pepper, and onion, and cook the vegetables until they're softened, about 8 to 10 minutes.

In a bowl, whisk the eggs with the cream, cheddar, salt, and pepper until combined. Whisk the vegetables into the egg mixture and pour it into a 9-inch pie plate.

Bake the quiche in the oven until it sets, about 40 to 45 minutes.

Cut the quiche into wedges and serve it immediately.

Nutritional Information
Per serving
Total Fat: 41.5 grams
Protein: 35 grams
Total Carbohydrates: 11.5 grams

BACON DEVILED EGGS

Makes 2 servings

4 bacon slices

8 large eggs

2 tablespoons sugar-free mayonnaise

1 teaspoon Dijon mustard

¼ teaspoon sea salt

¼ teaspoon ground black pepper

¼ teaspoon paprika

Cook the bacon in a skillet over medium heat until it's golden and crisp, about 8 to 10 minutes. Remove it from the skillet and finely chop the bacon.

Place the eggs in a pot and cover them with water. Bring the water to a boil and cook the eggs for 7 minutes. Remove the pot from the heat and allow the eggs to sit for 10 minutes. Remove the eggs from the hot water, place them in a colander, and rinse them with cold water until they are cooled.

Peel the eggs, cut them in half, and put the yolks in a bowl. Blend the yolks with the mayonnaise, Dijon, salt, and pepper until smooth. Stir in the bacon.

Pipe or spoon the yolk mixture into the egg halves. Dust them with paprika. Divide the deviled eggs between two plates and serve immediately.

Nutritional Information
Per serving (4 deviled eggs)
Total Fat: 35.5 grams
Protein: 31 grams
Total Carbohydrates: 1.5 grams

BUFFALO CHICKEN EGG MUFFINS

Makes 2 servings

3 tablespoons melted butter

6 large eggs

¼ teaspoon sea salt

¼ teaspoon ground black pepper

4 ounces chopped or shredded cooked chicken

2 tablespoons sugar-free hot sauce

2 teaspoons sliced chives

Preheat the oven to 375° F. Grease six cups of a muffin tin with the butter.

Whisk the eggs in a bowl with the salt and pepper until combined. Divide the chicken between the muffin cups and pour the eggs on top, ensuring there is an even amount in each one. Place the muffin tin on a baking sheet.

Bake the muffins until they set and are cooked through, about 25 to 30 minutes.

Remove the muffins from the pan and divide them between two plates.

Garnish the muffins with the hot sauce and chives, and serve immediately.

Nutritional Information

Per serving (3 muffins)

Total Fat: 34 grams

Protein: 35.5 grams

Total Carbohydrates: 1.5 grams

POACHED EGGS WITH HOLLANDAISE AND ASPARAGUS

Makes 2 servings

10 large eggs

10 asparagus spears

3 egg yolks

1 tablespoon lemon juice

1 teaspoon Dijon mustard

¼ teaspoon sea salt

¼ teaspoon ground black pepper

3 tablespoons melted butter, hot

Poach the eggs in a pot of simmering salted water until they're soft boiled, about 3 to 5 minutes.

Meanwhile, blanch the asparagus spears in a pot of boiling salted water until they're tender-crisp, about 8 to 10 minutes.

While the eggs and asparagus are cooking, blend the egg yolks with the lemon juice, Dijon, salt, and pepper in a blender until smooth. While continuing to blend the mixture, gradually add the hot, melted butter until the Hollandaise is thick and creamy.

Divide the eggs and asparagus between two plates, drizzle with the hollandaise, and serve immediately.

Nutritional Information
Per serving
Total Fat: 47.5 grams
Protein: 37.5 grams
Total Carbohydrates: 7.5 grams

RAINBOW VEGGIE AND BACON BREAKFAST HASH

Makes 2 servings

½ cup diced rutabaga

8 bacon slices, chopped

½ cup diced zucchini

½ orange, red, or yellow bell pepper, diced

1 teaspoon paprika

½ teaspoon onion powder

½ teaspoon garlic powder

½ teaspoon Italian seasoning

½ teaspoon sea salt

¼ teaspoon ground black pepper

1 tablespoon butter

8 large eggs

1 tablespoon finely chopped dill

Blanch the rutabaga in a small pot of boiling water for 6 to 8 minutes. Drain the rutabaga and set it aside.

Place the bacon in a nonstick skillet and heat it over medium heat; cook until the bacon is browned, about 8 minutes. Use a slotted spoon to move the bacon to a bowl and set it aside.

Return the skillet to medium heat. Add the rutabaga, zucchini, bell pepper, paprika, onion powder, garlic powder, Italian seasoning, salt, and pepper, and cook the vegetables until they are tender, about 10 minutes. Stir in the bacon and keep the hash warm.

Heat the butter in a separate nonstick skillet over medium heat. Whisk the eggs in a bowl until the mixture is smooth. Add the eggs to the skillet and let them cook without stirring for 1 minute. Start scrambling the eggs until they set in large, fluffy curds, about 3 to 4 minutes. Alternatively, cook them in any other style you prefer.

Divide the vegetables between two bowls and top each with half the eggs. Garnish the bowls with the dill and serve the hash immediately.

Nutritional Information
Per serving
Total Fat: 37 grams
Protein: 38 grams
Total Carbohydrates: 9 grams

CHICKEN SAUSAGE EGG WRAPS

Makes 2 servings

½ pound ground chicken

1 teaspoon fennel seeds

½ teaspoon onion powder

½ teaspoon sea salt

¼ teaspoon paprika

¼ teaspoon ground allspice

¼ teaspoon ground nutmeg

¼ teaspoon ground black pepper

2 tablespoons butter, divided

¼ cup shredded pecorino romano

6 large eggs, divided

In a bowl, gently knead the ground chicken with the fennel seeds, onion powder, salt, paprika, allspice, nutmeg, and black pepper until combined. Divide and shape the mixture into four patties.

Heat 1 tablespoon of the butter in a nonstick skillet over medium heat. Add the patties and cook them until they're golden and cooked through, about 5 minutes per side. Sprinkle the cheese on top of the patties, cover the skillet with a lid, and allow the cheese to melt, about 3 to 5 minutes.

Meanwhile, heat ½ tablespoon of the butter in a medium nonstick skillet over medium heat. Whisk the eggs, pour half the eggs in the skillet, cover them with a lid, and cook them until they set, about 3 to 5 minutes. Remove the omelette to a large cutting board or plate. Repeat the process to make a second omelette.

Place 2 sausage patties on top of each omelette and fold them to form wraps, fastening them with toothpicks if needed. Serve immediately.

Nutritional Information
Per serving
Total Fat: 40.5 grams
Protein: 39.5 grams
Total Carbohydrates: 2 grams

POACHED EGGS AND ZUCCHINI FRITTERS

Makes 2 servings

1 cup shredded zucchini

¼ cup shredded pecorino romano

11 eggs, divided

1 garlic clove, minced

½ teaspoon Italian seasoning

¼ teaspoon sea salt

¼ teaspoon ground black pepper

1 tablespoon butter

In a bowl, stir the zucchini with the cheese, 1 egg, garlic, Italian seasoning, sea salt, and pepper until combined.

Heat the butter in a large nonstick skillet over medium heat. Dollop the zucchini mixture into the skillet in four portions, flattening each slightly so they form a round. Cook until golden and crisp, about 5 minutes; flip and cook for another 5 minutes. Remove the zucchini fritters and divide them between two plates.

Meanwhile, poach the remaining 10 eggs in a pot of simmering water until they set but with the yolks still soft, about 3 to 5 minutes. Remove them with a slotted spoon. Alternatively, cook the eggs in another style if desired.

Serve the poached eggs with the fritters immediately.

Nutritional Information
Per serving
Total Fat: 35.5 grams
Protein: 35 grams
Total Carbohydrates: 4 grams

MUSHROOM SCRAMBLED EGGS WITH MÂCHE SALAD

Makes 2 servings

For the Scrambled Eggs

2 teaspoons butter
3 pounds sliced cremini mushrooms
½ teaspoon sea salt
¼ teaspoon finely ground black pepper
1 teaspoon dried thyme leaves
18 egg whites

For the Salad

6 cups mâche leaves (or you can use butter lettuce)
1 cup sliced radishes
8 green onions, sliced
¼ cup apple cider vinegar
2 tablespoons finely chopped tarragon
2 teaspoons Dijon mustard
¼ teaspoon sea salt
¼ teaspoon ground black pepper

For the scrambled eggs, heat the butter in a skillet over medium heat. Add the mushrooms, salt, pepper, and thyme, and cook until the mushrooms are golden brown, about 8 to 10 minutes.

Whisk the egg whites in a small bowl.

Pour the eggs into the skillet with the mushrooms and cook them, while stirring, until they're scrambled, about 3 to 5 minutes.

To make the salad, toss the mâche with the radishes and green onions until combined. In a small bowl, whisk the apple cider vinegar with the tarragon, Dijon, salt, and pepper until combined. Toss the dressing with the salad until it is well coated.

Divide the eggs and salad between two plates and serve immediately.

Nutritional Information
Per serving
Total Fat: 5 grams
Protein: 42.5 grams
Total Carbohydrates: 50.5 grams

LUNCH

SALMON CAKES AND ICEBERG SALAD

Makes 2 servings

10 ounces canned salmon, drained

4 tablespoons sugar-free mayonnaise, divided

1 teaspoon chopped capers

½ teaspoon lemon zest

½ teaspoon Italian seasoning

¼ teaspoon cayenne pepper

1 large egg white

1 tablespoon butter

2 cups shredded iceberg lettuce

¼ cup chopped cucumber

1 tablespoon sliced green onions

1 tablespoon apple cider vinegar

1 tablespoon chopped parsley

1 tablespoon chopped dill

Sea salt and ground black pepper, to taste

Mix the salmon in a bowl with 2 tablespoons of the mayonnaise, capers, lemon zest, Italian seasoning, and cayenne pepper until combined. Beat the egg white until stiff peaks form; gently fold it into the salmon mixture until combined. Divide and shape the mixture into four cakes.

Heat the butter in a skillet set over medium heat. Add the cakes, press them down with a spatula, and cook them until golden and heated through, about 4 to 6 minutes per side.

Divide the lettuce between two plates and top it with the cucumber and green onions. Place the salmon cakes on the side.

In a bowl, whisk the remaining mayonnaise with the vinegar, parsley, and dill, and salt and pepper to taste. Drizzle it over the salad and salmon cakes and serve immediately.

Nutritional Information
Per serving
Total Fat: 40 grams
Protein: 37.5 grams
Total Carbohydrates: 3 grams

TAMARI-SESAME BEEF LETTUCE WRAPS

Makes 2 servings

10 ounces flank or sirloin steak

2 tablespoons tamari

4 tablespoons sesame oil

1 tablespoon apple cider vinegar

2 teaspoons finely minced ginger

3 garlic cloves, minced

½ teaspoon sea salt

¼ teaspoon ground black pepper

8 Bibb or Boston lettuce leaves

2 tablespoons chopped cilantro

Thinly slice the steak into strips against the grain.

Whisk the tamari in a bowl with the sesame oil, vinegar, ginger, garlic, salt, and pepper until combined. Add the steak to the bowl and allow it to marinate for at least 30 minutes.

Heat a large skillet over medium-high heat. Add the steak mixture to the skillet and cook until the steak is just browned, about 3 to 5 minutes.

Divide the steak between the lettuce leaves and garnish them with cilantro.

Nutritional Information
Per serving
Total Fat: 39.5 grams
Protein: 33.5 grams
Total Carbohydrates: 4.5 grams

CHICKEN SHIRATAKI NOODLE SOUP

Makes 2 servings

6 tablespoons butter
2 garlic cloves, minced
4 cups chicken broth
8 ounces chicken breast, chopped into small cubes
1 carrot, chopped into small cubes
1 celery stalk, chopped into small cubes
2 teaspoons tamari
½ teaspoon dried thyme
½ teaspoon sea salt, or to taste
¼ teaspoon ground black pepper, or to taste
1 7-ounce package carb-free shirataki noodles such as Miracle Noodles

Heat the butter in a large pot over medium heat. Add the garlic and cook just until fragrant, about 1 minute.

Stir in the chicken broth, chicken, carrots, celery, tamari, thyme, salt, and pepper. Bring the mixture to a simmer and cook until the vegetables are soft, about 20 minutes.

Add the noodles and cook for another 5 minutes.

Divide the soup between two bowls and serve immediately.

Nutritional Information
Per serving
Total Fat: 37.5 grams
Protein: 37 grams
Total Carbohydrates: 7.5 grams

RAINBOW CHICKEN VEGETABLE SALAD

Makes 2 servings

2 teaspoons butter

6-ounce chicken breast

1 teaspoon sea salt, divided

½ teaspoon ground black pepper, divided

6 cups chopped romaine lettuce

2 large red bell peppers, cubed

2 large green bell peppers, cubed

4 cups sliced cucumber

2 cups shredded carrot

¼ cup sliced green onions

¼ cup torn dill leaves

¼ cup freshly squeezed lemon juice

¼ cup apple cider vinegar

1 tablespoon Dijon mustard

4 garlic cloves, minced

Heat the butter in a skillet over medium heat. Season the chicken with ½ teaspoon of salt and ¼ teaspoon of pepper. Add it to the skillet and cook until it's golden and cooked through, about 8 to 10 minutes per side. Remove the skillet from the heat and slice the chicken breast into strips.

While the chicken cooks, in a large bowl, toss the romaine with the bell peppers, cucumber slices, carrot, green onions, and dill until combined.

In a separate bowl, whisk the lemon juice with the vinegar, Dijon, garlic, and remaining salt and pepper until combined. Toss the salad with the dressing.

Divide the salad between two bowls, top it with the chicken, and serve immediately.

Nutritional Information
Per serving
Total Fat: 8 grams
Protein: 30 grams
Total Carbohydrates: 50.5 grams

SHIRATAKI FRIED RICE

Makes 2 servings

3 tablespoons butter

8 ounces pork loin chop, cubed

Sea salt, to taste

Ground black pepper, to taste

1 package shirataki rice

¼ cup sliced green onions

2 tablespoons tamari

4 garlic cloves, minced

1 teaspoon sesame oil

4 large eggs

Heat the butter in a skillet over medium heat.

Season the pork with salt and pepper to taste. Add it to the skillet and cook until it's golden and cooked through, about 8 to 10 minutes.

Add the shirataki rice, green onions, tamari, garlic, and sesame oil to the skillet. Cook, while stirring occasionally, until the mixture is heated through, about 10 minutes.

Whisk the eggs in a bowl. Move the rice to the side of the pan, add the eggs, and cook them until scrambled. Stir the eggs into the rice.

Divide the rice between two bowls and serve immediately.

Nutritional Information
Per serving
Total Fat: 38 grams
Protein: 38 grams
Total Carbohydrates: 8.5 grams

BURGERS ON ICEBERG LETTUCE BUNS

Makes 2 servings

For the Sauce

3 tablespoons sugar-free mayonnaise

1 tablespoon chopped dill pickle

1 tablespoon finely chopped onion

¼ teaspoon paprika

¼ teaspoon ground black pepper

For the Burgers

12 ounces ground beef

1 tablespoon Dijon mustard

1 tablespoon tamari

½ teaspoon sea salt

¼ teaspoon ground black pepper

1 teaspoon butter

4 iceberg lettuce leaves

To make the sauce, stir the mayonnaise, dill pickle, onion, paprika, and pepper until combined. Set aside.

For the burgers, gently knead the beef in a bowl with the Dijon mustard, tamari, salt, and pepper until combined. Divide the mixture into two portions and shape them into patties.

Heat the butter in a skillet over medium heat. Add the burgers and cook until cooked through, about 8 to 10 minutes per side.

Place each burger on an iceberg lettuce leaf, top them with the sauce, and cap them with another iceberg lettuce leaf. Serve immediately.

Nutritional Information

Per serving

Total Fat: 35.5 grams

Protein: 35 grams

Total Carbohydrates: 2 grams

BEEF KOFTA WITH GREEK SALAD AND TZATZIKI

Makes 2 servings

For the Beef Kofta

12 ounces ground beef

1 garlic clove, minced

½ teaspoon ground cumin

½ teaspoon ground coriander

¼ teaspoon sea salt

¼ teaspoon ground black pepper

4 bamboo skewers, soaked in water for at least 30 minutes and up to 12 hours

3 tablespoons olive oil

For the Tzatziki

¼ cup sheep milk yogurt

2 tablespoons shredded English cucumber

½ teaspoon finely chopped dill

1 teaspoon freshly squeezed lemon juice

½ garlic clove, minced

⅛ teaspoon sea salt

⅛ teaspoon freshly ground black pepper

For the Greek Salad

2 cups shredded iceberg lettuce

¼ cup chopped cucumber

6 grape or cherry tomatoes, halved

Make the beef kofta: Gently knead the ground beef in a bowl with the garlic, cumin, coriander, salt, and pepper until combined. Divide into four equal portions and press each portion around one of the bamboo skewers; repeat with the remaining ground beef mixture and skewers until you have four skewers. Brush the skewers with the olive oil.

Heat a large skillet over medium heat. Add the skewers and cook them, while turning, until golden and cooked through, about 10 to 12 minutes. Alternatively, you can cook the skewers on the grill if preferred.

Make the tzatziki: Stir the yogurt with the cucumber, dill, lemon juice, garlic, salt, and pepper until combined.

Make the Greek salad: Divide the lettuce between two plates and top them with the cucumber and tomatoes.

Arrange two skewers on top of each salad, drizzle them with the tzatziki, and serve immediately.

Nutritional Information
Per serving
Total Fat: 39 grams
Protein: 36 grams

SMOKED MACKEREL DIP

Makes 2 servings

8 ounces tinned smoked mackerel packed in oil

2 tablespoons butter, softened

1 teaspoon Dijon mustard

¼ teaspoon sea salt

⅛ teaspoon ground black pepper

20 cucumber slices

Mash the mackerel with a fork in a bowl with the butter, Dijon, salt, and pepper, until the mixture is combined and the mackerel is in small flakes. (Add 1 to 2 tablespoons of water if needed to create a wetter mixture.)

Divide the dip between two bowls, and serve with 10 cucumber slices each for dipping.

Nutritional Information
Per serving
Total Fat: 38 grams
Protein: 28 grams
Total Carbohydrates: 2 grams

LAMB BURGERS WITH TZATZIKI

Makes 2 servings

For the Burgers

10 ounces ground lamb

2 tablespoons finely chopped onion

1 tablespoon chopped parsley

1 tablespoon chopped mint

½ teaspoon ground cumin

½ teaspoon ground coriander

1 garlic clove, minced

½ teaspoon sea salt

¼ teaspoon freshly ground black pepper

2 tablespoons butter

4 iceberg lettuce leaves

For the Tzatziki

½ cup sheep's milk yogurt

¼ cup shredded English cucumber

1 teaspoon finely chopped dill

2 teaspoons freshly squeezed lemon juice

1 garlic clove, minced

¼ teaspoon sea salt

¼ teaspoon freshly ground black pepper

Make the burger patties: In a bowl, gently knead the lamb with the onion, parsley, mint, cumin, coriander, garlic, salt, and pepper until combined. Divide and shape the mixture into two patties and place them on a plate or small baking sheet. Refrigerate the patties until they set, about 30 minutes.

Make the tzatziki: Stir the yogurt with the cucumber, dill, lemon juice, garlic, salt, and pepper until combined. Put the tzatziki in the fridge until you're ready to use it.

Heat the butter in a skillet over medium heat until it's melted and sizzling. Add the patties and cook them until they're golden on both sides and cooked through, about 8 to 10 minutes per side.

Serve each burger between two pieces of iceberg lettuce and topped with the tzatziki.

Nutritional Information
Per serving
Total Fat: 40.5 grams
Protein: 34 grams
Total Carbohydrates: 8 grams

CHIPOTLE SALMON WITH CILANTRO-LIME SLAW

Makes 2 servings

For the Salmon
2 8-ounce salmon fillets
1 tablespoon olive oil
1 teaspoon chipotle chili powder (or regular chili powder)
Salt and pepper, to taste

For the Cilantro-Lime Slaw
2 tablespoons freshly squeezed lime juice
4 tablespoons olive oil
½ teaspoon sea salt
¼ teaspoon ground black pepper
1 cup shredded green cabbage
2 tablespoons chopped cilantro

Preheat the oven to 375° F. Line a small baking sheet with parchment paper.

Arrange the salmon fillets on the baking sheet and coat them with olive oil, chili powder, and salt and pepper to taste. Roast the fillets in the oven until the salmon flakes easily with a fork, about 15 to 20 minutes.

Recipes

Make the slaw: Whisk the lime juice with the olive oil, salt, and pepper until combined. Toss the cabbage with the cilantro and dressing until combined.

Divide the salmon and slaw between two plates and serve them immediately.

Nutritional Information
Per serving
Total Fat: 36 grams
Protein: 42.5 grams
Total Carbohydrates: 5.5 grams

MEATLOAF MUFFINS AND RUTABAGA MASH

Makes 2 servings

For the Meatloaf Muffins

12 ounces ground beef

1 large egg

1 tablespoon Dijon mustard

1 teaspoon Italian seasoning

½ teaspoon sea salt

½ teaspoon ground black pepper

For the Rutabaga Mash

1 cup cubed rutabaga

4 tablespoons butter

½ teaspoon sea salt

¼ teaspoon black pepper

Preheat the oven to 375° F.

In a bowl, knead the beef with the egg, Dijon, Italian seasoning, salt, and pepper until combined. Divide the mixture into four portions, and press each one into a cup of a muffin tin. Place the tin on a baking sheet and bake the muffins until they are cooked through and a meat thermometer reaches 165° F, about 30 to 40 minutes.

231

Place the rutabaga cubes in a pot and cover them with water. Boil the rutabaga until it is soft, about 50 to 60 minutes.

Drain the rutabaga and return it to the pot. Add the butter, salt, and pepper, and mash until smooth.

Divide the meatloaf muffins and rutabaga between two plates, and serve immediately.

Nutritional Information
Per serving
Total Fat: 42.5 grams
Protein: 37.5 grams
Total Carbohydrates: 7 grams

WARM BACON, EGG, AND ASPARAGUS SALAD

Makes 2 servings

8 large eggs

16 asparagus spears, woody stems removed

6 bacon slices, sliced into thick strips, cut into 1-inch pieces

2 tablespoons apple cider vinegar

1 tablespoon olive oil

1 teaspoon Dijon mustard

¼ teaspoon sea salt

¼ teaspoon ground black pepper

Place the eggs in a pot and cover them with water. Bring the water to a boil and then reduce to a simmer, and simmer the eggs for 7 minutes. Remove the pot from the heat and allow it to sit for 10 minutes. Remove the eggs and rinse them with cold water to stop the cooking process. Peel and chop the eggs.

Blanch the asparagus in a pot of simmering salted water until it's tender-crisp, about 6 minutes. Drain the spears and run cold water over them to stop the cooking process.

Cook the bacon in a skillet over medium heat until browned and crisp, about 8 to 10 minutes. Use a slotted spoon to move the bacon to a paper-towel-lined plate.

Whisk the vinegar, olive oil, Dijon, salt, and pepper into the bacon fat.

Toss the asparagus and bacon with the dressing and divide it between two plates. Top each portion with the eggs and serve immediately.

Nutritional Information
Per serving
Total Fat: 35 grams
Protein: 36.5 grams
Total Carbohydrates: 7 grams

PASTA CARBONARA

Makes 2 servings

3 large eggs
½ cup shredded pecorino romano, divided
½ teaspoon sea salt
½ teaspoon ground black pepper
1 tablespoon olive oil
4 ounces bacon, chopped
8 ounces shirataki noodles, drained and rinsed
1 tablespoon chopped parsley

Whisk the eggs in a bowl with ⅓ cup of cheese and the salt and pepper until combined.

Heat the olive oil in a skillet over medium heat. Add the bacon and cook until browned and crisp, about 8 to 10 minutes. Add the noodles and stir-fry the noodles and bacon until the noodles are warmed through, about 3 minutes.

Remove the noodles from the heat; add the egg mixture and toss until a creamy sauce is formed.

Divide the mixture between two bowls, sprinkle with the remaining cheese and parsley, and serve immediately. Add black pepper to taste.

Nutritional Information
Per serving
Total Fat: 40 grams
Protein: 33 grams
Total Carbohydrates: 1.5 grams

DINNER

SLOW-COOKED LEMON-HERB CHICKEN AND CARROTS

Makes 2 servings

⅓ cup softened butter

1 tablespoon finely grated lemon zest

1 tablespoon freshly squeezed lemon juice

2 garlic cloves, minced

1 teaspoon chopped rosemary

1 teaspoon chopped thyme

½ teaspoon sea salt

¼ teaspoon ground black pepper

2 large carrots, peeled and sliced

1 cup chicken broth

2 10-ounce chicken legs

Cream the butter with the lemon zest, lemon juice, garlic, rosemary, thyme, salt, and pepper until combined.

Place the carrots in the bowl of a slow cooker and add the chicken broth.

Rub the chicken legs in the butter mixture and place them on top of the carrots.

Cook on high until the carrots and chicken are cooked through, about 4 to 5 hours.

Tip: If you would like the chicken to have more color, once it is cooked you can place it on a baking sheet under the broiler for 5 to 10 minutes, or until it is golden brown.

Nutritional Information
Per serving
Total Fat: 48.5 grams
Protein: 72 grams
Total Carbohydrates: 8 grams

COD AND BACON SOUP

Makes 2 servings

1 tablespoon butter

6 bacon slices, sliced into thick strips, cut into 1-inch pieces

¼ onion, diced

1 garlic clove, minced

½ teaspoon paprika

½ teaspoon sea salt

¼ teaspoon ground black pepper

⅛ teaspoon cayenne pepper, or more to taste

4 cups seafood stock or clam broth

8 ounces fresh or frozen cod (thawed), cut into 1-inch chunks

½ cup heavy cream

2 tablespoons freshly squeezed lemon juice

1 tablespoon chopped parsley

Heat the butter in a large pot over medium heat. Cook the bacon until golden and crispy, about 8 to 10 minutes. Remove the bacon with a slotted spoon, leaving the fat behind, and set it aside.

Return the pot with the bacon fat to medium heat. Add the onion, garlic, paprika, salt, pepper, and cayenne, and cook the onion until it is soft and translucent, about 10 minutes.

Add the seafood stock and bring it to a simmer.

Add the cod to the pot with the bacon and simmer the mixture until the cod is cooked, about 5 to 7 minutes.

Stir in the heavy cream, lemon juice, and parsley. Simmer for an additional 5 minutes until heated through.

Divide the soup between two bowls and serve immediately.

Nutritional Information
Per serving
Total Fat: 36.5 grams
Protein: 33 grams
Total Carbohydrates: 7.5 grams

SAUCY BEEF AND MUSHROOM STEW

Makes 2 servings

12 ounces stewing beef

1 cup sliced cremini mushrooms

1 carrot, chopped

1 celery stalk, chopped

¼ onion, diced

3 cups beef stock

1 tablespoon apple cider vinegar

2 teaspoons tamari

1 teaspoon chopped rosemary

½ teaspoon dried thyme

½ teaspoon sea salt

¼ teaspoon ground black pepper

Combine the beef, mushrooms, carrots, celery, and onion in a slow cooker. Add in the beef stock, vinegar, tamari, rosemary, thyme, salt, and pepper, and stir until combined.

Cook on high until the beef and vegetables are tender, about 6 to 8 hours.

Divide between two bowls and serve immediately.

Tip: If you would like a thicker stew, whisk in about ½ teaspoon of xanthan gum toward the end of the cooking time so that it can thicken. Feel free to adjust the quantity of xanthan gum, depending on the thickness you prefer.

Nutritional Information
Per serving
Total Fat: 35.5 grams
Protein: 35.5 grams
Total Carbohydrates: 8 grams

KETO CHICKEN PICCATA

Makes 2 servings

2 6-ounce chicken breasts, sliced in half horizontally

½ teaspoon sea salt

¼ teaspoon ground black pepper

3 tablespoons cold butter, divided

3 tablespoons olive oil

¼ cup freshly squeezed lemon juice

¼ cup chicken broth

2 tablespoons capers

Sea salt and ground black pepper, to taste

2 tablespoons chopped parsley

Season the chicken with the salt and pepper. Heat 1 tablespoon of butter and the olive oil in a nonstick skillet over medium heat. Add the chicken and cook it until it's golden on both sides and cooked through, about 10 to 15 minutes. Remove the chicken and set it aside.

Add the lemon juice, chicken broth, capers, and salt and pepper to the skillet, and bring to a simmer. Stir in the remaining butter. Add the chicken, reduce the heat to low, and allow it to warm through for 5 minutes.

Divide the chicken piccata and sauce between two plates and garnish with parsley.

Nutritional Information
Per serving
Total Fat: 42.5 grams
Protein: 39 grams
Total Carbohydrates: 2.5 grams

CHICKEN SKEWERS WITH ZUCCHINI AND BELL PEPPERS

Makes 2 servings

12 ounces chicken breast, cut into 1-inch cubes

½ red, orange, yellow, or green bell pepper, cut into 1-inch cubes

½ zucchini, sliced into ½-inch-thick rounds and cut into half-moons if large

3 tablespoons olive oil

2 tablespoons freshly squeezed lemon juice

2 teaspoons dried oregano

½ teaspoon paprika

½ teaspoon onion powder

3 garlic cloves, minced

½ teaspoon salt

¼ teaspoon red pepper flakes

4 large bamboo skewers, soaked in water for at least 30 minutes and up to 12 hours

½ lemon

Place the chicken in a dish and the vegetables in another dish.

In a bowl, whisk the olive oil with the lemon juice, oregano, paprika, onion powder, garlic, salt, and red pepper flakes until combined. Pour half of the mixture over the chicken and half over the vegetables, allowing everything to marinate for at least 30 minutes.

Thread the chicken and vegetables onto the skewers, alternating the chicken with the peppers and zucchini.

Heat a grill to medium heat. Add the skewers and cook, while turning, until the chicken is golden and cooked through, about 15 to 20 minutes. Meanwhile, grill the lemon half face down until it chars slightly, about 5 to 10 minutes.

Squeeze some lemon over the skewers and divide them between two plates; serve immediately.

Nutritional Information

Per serving (2 skewers)

Total Fat: 36.5 grams

Protein: 37 grams

Total Carbohydrates: 9.5 grams

OREGANO-MUSTARD SALMON WITH BROCCOLI

Makes 2 servings

2 tablespoons Dijon mustard

6 tablespoons melted butter, divided

½ teaspoon dried oregano

2 garlic cloves, minced

¼ teaspoon sea salt

¼ teaspoon freshly ground black pepper

14 ounces salmon fillets, fresh or frozen (thawed)

2 cups broccoli florets

Preheat the oven to 350° F.

Mix the Dijon in a bowl with 2 tablespoons of butter and the oregano, garlic, salt, and pepper. Stir until combined.

Rub the salmon with the mustard mixture on both sides, and place the fillets on a parchment paper–lined baking sheet. Bake until the salmon flakes easily with a fork, about 15 to 20 minutes.

Meanwhile, cook the broccoli in a pot of boiling salted water until tender-crisp, about 6 to 8 minutes. Drain the broccoli and toss it with the remaining melted butter.

Divide the salmon and broccoli between two plates and serve immediately.

Nutritional Information
Per serving
Total Fat: 38.5 grams
Protein: 39 grams
Total Carbohydrates: 5 grams

CRISPY FISH AND TARTAR SAUCE

Makes 2 servings

For the Fish

10 ounces firm-fleshed white fish, such as cod or halibut

1 large egg

1 ounce pork rinds, finely crushed

2 tablespoons butter

For the Tartar Sauce

¼ cup sugar-free mayonnaise

1 tablespoon finely chopped dill pickle

1 teaspoon white wine vinegar

1 teaspoon finely chopped capers

½ teaspoon sugar-free grainy mustard

1 pinch sea salt

1 pinch ground black pepper

Cut the fish into four to six pieces. Beat the egg in a bowl. Place the pork rinds in another bowl. Dip each piece of fish in the egg followed by the pork rinds until coated.

Heat the butter in a skillet over medium heat. Add the fish and cook the pieces until they are golden, about 5 to 8 minutes. Turn the pieces over and cook them for another 5 to 8 minutes or until they are cooked through.

Make the tartar sauce: Whisk the mayonnaise with the dill pickle, vinegar, capers, mustard, salt, and pepper until well combined.

Divide the fish between two plates and serve the tartar sauce on the side.

Nutritional Information
Per serving
Total Fat: 36.5 grams
Protein: 30.5 grams
Total Carbohydrates: 1 gram

SKILLET CHICKEN FAJITAS

Makes 2 servings

5 tablespoons butter

12 ounces chicken breast, sliced

1 medium red, green, orange, or green bell pepper, sliced into strips

½ onion, sliced

1 teaspoon chili powder

½ teaspoon cumin

½ teaspoon onion powder

½ teaspoon garlic powder

½ teaspoon salt

1 pinch cayenne pepper, or more to taste

¼ cup sour cream

Heat the butter in a skillet. Add the chicken, bell pepper, onion, chili powder, cumin, onion powder, garlic powder, salt, and cayenne, and cook until the chicken is cooked through and the bell pepper is tender, about 10 to 15 minutes.

Divide between two bowls, garnish with the sour cream, and serve immediately.

Nutritional Information
Per serving
Total Fat: 39.5 grams
Protein: 41 grams
Total Carbohydrates: 9 grams

KETO FISH CHOWDER

Makes 2 servings

6 bacon slices, chopped

½ cup finely chopped cauliflower florets

½ cup chopped onion

1 celery stalk, chopped

1 garlic clove, minced

1 cup chicken broth

1 cup water

1 cup heavy cream

½ teaspoon sea salt

¼ teaspoon ground black pepper

12 ounces cod or halibut, cut into 1-inch cubes

1 tablespoon finely chopped parsley

Cook the bacon in a large pot over medium heat until it's golden, about 8 to 10 minutes. Remove the bacon with a slotted spoon and set aside. Deglaze the pot with some water if needed.

Add the cauliflower, onion, celery, and garlic to the pot and cook the vegetables until the onions are translucent, about 10 minutes. Stir in the chicken broth, water, cream, salt, and pepper; bring to a simmer and allow the chowder to cook until the cauliflower and celery are tender, about 15 to 20 minutes.

Stir in the fish and bacon, and simmer the chowder for another 5 minutes.

Divide the chowder between two bowls, garnish with the parsley, and serve immediately.

Nutritional Information
Per serving
Total Fat: 31.5 grams
Protein: 44.5 grams
Total Carbohydrates: 7.5 grams

POACHED CHICKEN BREAST WITH CREAMY BASIL SAUCE AND ASPARAGUS

Makes 2 servings

1 cup basil leaves

1 tablespoon lemon juice

1 teaspoon lemon zest

1 garlic clove, minced

½ teaspoon sea salt

¼ teaspoon freshly ground black pepper

⅓ cup olive oil

2 6-ounce chicken breasts

16 asparagus spears, woody stems removed

Using an upright blender or food processor, blend the basil with the lemon juice, lemon zest, garlic, salt, and pepper until the basil is coarsely chopped. Continue blending while adding the olive oil in a slow drizzle until a sauce is formed.

Place the chicken breasts in a pot of cold salted water. Bring it to a boil; then, cover and reduce it to a simmer, allowing the chicken to poach until cooked through, about 10 to 12 minutes.

Blanch the asparagus in a pot of boiling salted water until tender-crisp, about 6 to 8 minutes.

Serve the chicken drizzled with the basil sauce alongside the asparagus.

Nutritional Information

Per serving
Total Fat: 40 grams
Protein: 42 grams
Total Carbohydrates: 6.5 grams

KETO TEXAS CHILI

Makes 2 servings

4 tablespoons butter

12 ounces beef roast, such as chuck roast, cubed

2 cups beef bone broth

1 tablespoon apple cider vinegar

1 tablespoon chili powder

1 tablespoon chipotle sauce, from a can of chipotle chilis

½ teaspoon dried oregano

½ teaspoon sea salt

¼ teaspoon ground black pepper

¼ cup sour cream

Heat the butter in a large skillet over medium heat. Add half the beef and cook it until browned, about 5 minutes. Remove the beef to a plate and repeat the process to brown the other half.

Combine the beef, beef stock, apple cider vinegar, chili powder, chipotle sauce, oregano, salt, and pepper in a slow cooker. Cook on high until the beef is tender, about 6 to 8 hours.

Divide the chili between two bowls, garnish them with the sour cream, and serve immediately.

Nutritional Information
Per serving
Total Fat: 40.5 grams
Protein: 38 grams
Total Carbohydrates: 7.5 grams

KETO BEEF STROGANOFF

Makes 2 servings

2 tablespoons butter

12 ounces sirloin steak, sliced into strips

Sea salt and ground black pepper, to taste

1 cup sliced cremini mushrooms

1 garlic clove, minced

½ teaspoon dried thyme

½ teaspoon sea salt

¼ teaspoon ground black pepper

½ cup beef broth

¼ cup sour cream

1 tablespoon finely chopped dill

Heat the butter in a skillet over medium-high heat. Season the steak with salt and pepper to taste, add it to the skillet, and cook until golden, about 3 to 5 minutes. Remove the steak and set it aside.

Add the mushrooms, garlic, thyme, salt, and pepper, and cook them until golden, about 8 to 10 minutes.

Stir in the beef broth and steak, and bring to a simmer for 3 minutes. Stir in the sour cream.

Divide the beef stroganoff between two bowls, garnish with the dill, and serve immediately.

Nutritional Information

Per serving

Total Fat: 38 grams

Protein: 36 grams

Total Carbohydrates: 3 grams

THAI RED CURRY CHICKEN SKEWERS AND SALAD

Makes 2 servings

For the Chicken Skewers

12 ounces chicken breast

2 tablespoons sugar-free, keto-friendly Thai red curry paste

3 tablespoons olive oil

1 tablespoon tamari

1 tablespoon freshly squeezed lime juice

1 teaspoon finely grated ginger

1 garlic clove, minced

4 bamboo skewers, soaked in water

For the Salad

2 tablespoons olive oil

1 tablespoon freshly squeezed lime juice

1 tablespoon apple cider vinegar

¼ teaspoon sea salt

¼ teaspoon ground black pepper

2 cups shredded iceberg lettuce

¼ cup julienne red bell pepper

1 tablespoon roughly chopped cilantro

Cut the chicken into 1-inch cubes.

In a bowl, whisk the curry paste with the olive oil, tamari, lime juice, ginger, and garlic until well combined. Add the chicken to the bowl and stir to coat the cubes. Allow the chicken to marinate in the fridge for at least 30 minutes.

Thread the chicken onto the skewers.

Heat a large skillet or grill pan over medium heat. Add the chicken skewers and cook them, turning them occasionally, until the chicken is golden brown and cooked through, about 12 to 15 minutes. Alternatively, cook the skewers on a grill over medium heat.

To make the dressing, whisk the olive oil with the lime juice, vinegar, salt, and pepper until combined.

Divide the lettuce between two plates and top it with the red bell pepper and cilantro. Drizzle the salad with the dressing.

Place the chicken skewers on top of the salad and serve immediately.

Nutritional Information
Per serving (2 skewers)
Total Fat: 40.5 grams
Protein: 40 grams
Total Carbohydrates: 6.5 grams

Metabolic Flex Day (Keto Flex) Recipes

BREAKFAST

EGG WHITE AND VEGETABLE BREAKFAST SKILLET

Make 2 servings

2 teaspoons butter, divided

1 ½ red, orange, or yellow bell peppers, cut into cubes

3 small zucchini, sliced into half-moons

3 pounds cremini mushrooms, sliced

24 Brussels sprouts, shredded

6 garlic cloves, minced

2 teaspoons paprika

2 teaspoons Italian seasoning

½ teaspoon sea salt, or to taste

¼ teaspoon ground black pepper, or to taste

20 large egg whites

Heat 1 teaspoon of the butter in a large skillet over medium heat. Add the bell peppers, zucchini, mushrooms, Brussels sprouts, garlic, paprika, Italian seasoning, salt, and pepper, and cook until the vegetables are tender, about 10 to 15 minutes.

Whisk the egg whites in a bowl with salt and pepper to taste.

Heat the remaining butter in a nonstick skillet over medium heat. Add the egg whites and cook until scrambled, about 3 to 5 minutes.

Divide the vegetable mixture between two plates, top with the eggs, and serve immediately.

Nutritional Information

Per serving

Total Fat: 6.5 grams

Protein: 46.5 grams

Total Carbohydrates: 60.5 grams

EGG AND SQUASH-STUFFED BELL PEPPERS

Makes 2 servings

5 large red bell peppers

4 teaspoons butter

1 pound butternut squash, peeled and cut into small cubes

1 teaspoon Italian seasoning

3 garlic cloves, minced

½ teaspoon sea salt

¼ teaspoon ground black pepper

14 large egg whites

Preheat the oven to 350° F.

Cut the bell peppers in half vertically and remove the stems and inner membrane and seeds. Set the peppers in a baking dish with the hollow side facing up.

Heat the butter in a skillet over medium heat. Add the squash, Italian seasoning, garlic, salt, and pepper, and cook until the squash can be pierced with a fork, about 15 minutes.

Divide the squash between the bell pepper halves. Cover tightly and bake until tender, about 1 hour.

Whisk the egg whites in a bowl, divide between the bell pepper halves, cover, and continue to bake until the eggs set, about 15 minutes.

Nutritional Information
Per serving
Total Fat: 9 grams
Protein: 32 grams
Total Carbohydrates: 42.5 grams

LUNCH

THAI-INSPIRED STEAK SALAD

Makes 2 servings

For the Steak

6 ounces flank steak

3 tablespoons tamari

3/4 teaspoon sea salt

¼ teaspoon ground black pepper

For the Salad

4 cups chopped romaine lettuce or green leaf lettuce

4 red, orange, yellow, or green bell peppers, thinly sliced

4 English cucumbers, sliced into half-moons

1 cup torn mint leaves

1 cup torn cilantro leaves

2 Thai chili peppers, thinly sliced

For the Dressing

6 tablespoons freshly squeezed lime juice

2 tablespoons tamari

1 teaspoon olive oil

2 garlic cloves, minced

¼ teaspoon red pepper flakes, or more to taste

¼ teaspoon sea salt

¼ teaspoon ground black pepper

Rub the steak with the tamari, salt, and pepper. Put it on a plate and allow it to marinate in the fridge for at least 30 minutes.

Heat a cast iron skillet over medium heat. Add the steak and cook until medium rare, about 4 minutes per side (alternatively, cook it to desired doneness). Remove it from the heat and allow it to rest for at least 5 minutes before slicing it.

Meanwhile, to make the salad, toss the lettuce with the bell peppers, cucumber, mint, cilantro, and Thai chili peppers until combined.

In a separate bowl, whisk the lime juice with the tamari, olive oil, garlic, red pepper flakes, salt, and pepper until combined.

Toss the salad with the steak and dressing, divide between two plates, and serve immediately.

Nutritional Information
Per serving
Total Fat: 8.5 grams
Protein: 33 grams
Total Carbohydrates: 51 grams

BUFFALO CHICKEN SOUP

Makes 2 servings

1 teaspoon butter

6 ounces chicken breast, cubed

4 red bell peppers, sliced

4 green bell peppers, sliced

1 medium onion, sliced

1 teaspoon paprika

3 garlic cloves, minced

½ teaspoon sea salt

½ teaspoon ground black pepper

1 cup chicken bone broth

3 tablespoons sugar-free cayenne pepper hot sauce

¼ cup chopped chives

Melt the butter in a saucepan over medium heat. Add the chicken, bell peppers, onion, paprika, garlic, salt, and pepper, and cook until the chicken is golden and the onions are translucent, about 10 to 12 minutes.

Add 3 cups water, the chicken broth, and the hot sauce, and bring the soup to a simmer. Cook until the vegetables are tender and the soup is heated through, about 10 minutes.

Divide the soup between two large bowls, garnish with the chives, and serve immediately.

Nutritional Information
Per serving
Total Fat: 9 grams
Protein: 39 grams
Total Carbohydrates: 51.5 grams

KETO MINESTRONE SOUP

Makes 2 servings

8 ounces lean ground beef

1 medium onion, chopped

2 teaspoons Italian seasoning

4 garlic cloves, minced

1 teaspoon sea salt

½ teaspoon ground black pepper

5 cups small cauliflower florets

3 celery stalks, cubed

4 large carrots, peeled and cubed

3 medium zucchini, cubed

¼ cup chopped parsley

Heat a large pot on the stove over medium heat. Add the ground beef, onion, Italian seasoning, garlic, salt, and pepper, and cook until the ground beef is browned, about 8 to 10 minutes.

Add the cauliflower, celery, carrots, zucchini, and at least 4 cups water. Bring to a simmer and cook the vegetables until they are tender (adding more water if needed), about 30 to 40 minutes. Taste and adjust the seasonings if needed.

Divide the soup between two large bowls, garnish with the parsley, and serve immediately.

Nutritional Information

Per serving

Total Fat: 10 grams

Protein: 35 grams

Total Carbohydrates: 47 grams

DINNER

CHICKEN AND VEGETABLE STIR-FRY

Makes 2 servings

1 teaspoon butter

6 ounces chicken breast, cut into cubes

1 pound sliced cremini mushrooms

8 cups small broccoli florets

4 red bell peppers, cut into strips

⅓ cup tamari

4 garlic cloves, minced

1 tablespoon finely minced ginger

½ teaspoon red pepper flakes

½ teaspoon sea salt

¼ cup chopped cilantro

Heat the butter in a large skillet. Add the chicken and cook until it's golden and cooked through, about 10 to 12 minutes. Remove and set aside.

Return the skillet to medium heat. Add the mushrooms, broccoli, and bell peppers, and cook the vegetables until they're golden, about 10 minutes. Add ¼ cup water, cover the skillet, and steam the vegetables until the broccoli is tender, about 5 minutes. Remove the lid and cook until the water has steamed off.

Whisk the tamari with the garlic, ginger, red pepper flakes, and salt.

Stir the sauce and chicken into the vegetables and cook until heated through, about 3 minutes.

Divide the stir-fry between two plates, garnish with the cilantro, and serve immediately.

Nutritional Information
Per serving
Total Fat: 7 grams
Protein: 45 grams
Total Carbohydrates: 49.5 grams

LEMONY COD AND VEGETABLE BAKE

Makes 2 servings

48 asparagus spears, woody ends removed

4 medium zucchini, sliced

4 yellow summer squash, sliced

2 3-ounce cod fillets

¼ cup freshly squeezed lemon juice

2 teaspoons melted butter

½ teaspoon sea salt

¼ teaspoon ground black pepper

2 tablespoons chopped parsley

Preheat the oven to 350° F.

Arrange the asparagus, zucchini, and summer squash in a large baking dish. Place the cod on top and season everything with the lemon juice, butter, salt, and pepper.

Cover tightly and bake until the fish is cooked and the vegetables are tender, about 30 to 40 minutes.

Divide between two plates and sprinkle with parsley.

Nutritional Information
Per serving
Total Fat: 6.5 grams
Protein: 35.5 grams
Total Carbohydrates: 49 grams

CHIPOTLE-DUSTED COD AND ZESTY LIME SLAW

Makes 2 servings

6 cups shredded red cabbage

6 cups shredded green cabbage

1 red onion, finely chopped

1 cup chopped cilantro

2 jalapeños, finely chopped

½ cup freshly squeezed lime juice

1 teaspoon sea salt, divided

½ teaspoon ground black pepper, divided

2 5-ounce cod fillets

½ teaspoon chipotle chili powder

2 teaspoons butter

In a large bowl, toss the cabbage, red onion, cilantro, jalapeños, lime juice, ½ teaspoon sea salt, and ¼ teaspoon ground black pepper until combined. Taste and adjust the salt and pepper if needed. Set the slaw aside.

Season the cod with the remaining salt and pepper and the chipotle powder.

Heat the butter in a skillet over medium heat. Add the fish and cook until golden and cooked through, about 4 to 5 minutes per side.

Divide the slaw between two bowls, top it with the cod, and serve immediately.

Nutritional Information
Per serving
Total Fat: 4.5 grams
Protein: 35.5 grams
Total Carbohydrates: 55 grams

AFTERWORD

I want to share something surprising with you. I never set out to become a world leader in metabolic health; it grew out of my own journey from pain to purpose. I spent much of my life feeling trapped by metabolic issues and ultimately lost my father to complications from diabetes. Often, our greatest pain can lead us to our most meaningful purpose, so I'm now passionate about educating people on how to remove the obstacles that are preventing their bodies from healing naturally.

I've been deeply discouraged by the state of the conventional medical industry. While I'm grateful for the dedicated doctors and health practitioners working tirelessly within the system, I'm also disheartened by how broken that system is. It's time we take control of our own health. This book is the manual I wish I'd had when I was struggling with obesity and when my father was battling debilitating diabetes. When you know better, you can do better. I am on a mission to help one billion people achieve metabolic freedom —a feat that has never been accomplished before. My commitment is driven by a desire to help others break free from the limitations of this metabolic disease, in honor of my father. If you'd like to learn more about my coaching programs, I invite you to visit www.benazadi.com to learn more.

You now have the exact steps to tap into your innate intelligence for deep healing. The keys to the health kingdom are in your hands. If you still have doubts or self-limiting beliefs about achieving metabolic freedom, let me share a story with you.

In South Africa, it's common for baby elephants to be put to work as soon as they can walk. After a long day of labor, chains are placed around their ankles and staked into the ground overnight to keep them in place. As the sun rises, the chains are removed, and the elephants return to work. At night, the baby elephant tries to break free, longing for freedom, but it's too small and weak to escape the chains. After several weeks of trying, the elephant gives up. Eventually, that baby elephant grows into a powerful adult, capable of pulling five times its own body weight and even moving loaded railroad carts. Yet, each night, the same chains are placed around its ankles, and the elephant doesn't even attempt to escape, despite being fully capable of breaking free. The elephant has been conditioned to believe that when those chains are around its ankles, it is trapped.

What mental chains have been placed on you? Think of this quote from a pioneer in spiritual and self-development growth, Vernon Howard: "You cannot escape a prison if you don't know you are in one."

My hope is that *Metabolic Freedom* has made you aware of the chains that have held you back. This book is designed to play a vital role in addressing the epidemic of disease in the world. As more people embrace the principles outlined here, I envision a future where we all unite in health, take responsibility for our well-being, and achieve lasting healing. I truly believe that the ancient healing strategies I've shared with you can dramatically transform the metabolic health of the world.

I dream of a time when we all recognize that the greatest physician who ever lived resides within our own bodies. The time to begin this journey is now. As Paulo Coelho said, "One day you will wake up and there won't be any more time to do the things you've always wanted. Do it now." Take pride in this newfound empowerment and in the growth you will experience. Support others who are on the same path. Turn "someday" into "day one." This is your day one. I am rooting for you every step of the way. I have an abundance of gratitude—vitamin G—for you. I love you, and I'm cheering you on with all my heart.

APPENDIX A

Glossary of Most-Used Metabolic Terms

Here are a few terms that you will see referenced often among metabolic freedom users worldwide. It's good to familiarize yourself with them before you start your journey.

Autophagy (aw-TAH-fuh-jee): A process by which a cell breaks down and destroys old, damaged, or abnormal proteins and other substances in its cytoplasm (the fluid inside a cell). The broken-down products are then recycled for important cell functions, especially during periods of fasting. This can occur after 16 to 18 hours of fasting but can happen sooner or later depending on your metabolic health.

Basal metabolic rate (BMR): The rate at which the body uses energy while at rest to keep vital functions going, such as breathing and keeping warm. In short, this is the number of calories your body would burn if you sat on the couch all day. Overweight people who have calorically restricted typically have lower basal metabolic rates.

Blood sugar: The blood glucose level is the amount of glucose in the blood. Glucose is a sugar that comes from the foods we eat, and it's also formed and stored inside the body via liver and muscle cells. Healthy blood sugar should be between 70 and 90 mg/dL (milligrams per deciliter) when in a fasted state.

Breaking a fast: The term *breakfast* simply means you are "breaking your fast" from not eating food overnight. We also use this term to refer to a food or drink that raises blood sugar and starts the digestive system, thus turning off the healing benefits of being in a fasted state. In short, this means you have pulled yourself out of a fast and into a fed state.

Eating window: The period throughout your day when you are eating. You would eat all your meals and snacks within a particular window of time each day. This timeframe can vary according to the person's preference and the plan they choose to follow.

Fasting window: The period throughout your day when you are not eating or drinking beverages that raise glucose. Any food or drink that raises blood sugar and starts the digestive process will pull you out of your fasted window.

Fat-adapted: Fat adaptation can occur to different degrees and across a spectrum dependent on the degree of carb restriction. This usually occurs generally when carbohydrates are restricted to under 50 total grams per day, over a period of seven days. You are fat-adapted when you have shifted away from primarily burning sugar (glucose) to burning fat (ketones).

Insulin: A hormone made by the islet cells of the pancreas. Insulin controls the amount of sugar in the blood by moving it into the cells, where it can be used by the body for energy. Insulin is the primary fat-storage hormone.

Insulin resistance: Insulin resistance is when cells in your muscles, fat, and liver don't respond well to insulin and can't easily take up glucose from your blood. As a result, your pancreas makes more insulin to help glucose enter your cells. A more accurate term would be *hyperinsulinemia*. If not corrected, over time this can lead to prediabetes, and eventually diabetes.

Intermittent fasting (IF): Going without food for 12 to 20 hours.

Keto-adapted: Keto adaptation represents a more comprehensive reshaping of many physiologic systems. Keto adaptation only happens when carbs are restricted to a point that induces sustained nutritional ketosis. This process takes longer than fat adaptation. It is estimated to take 6 to 12 weeks.

Keto flexing: Going in and out of ketosis after you've taught your body to be a fat burner. We also call this Metabolic Flexing. Some people call this carbohydrate cycling or keto cycling.

Ketones: A by-product of fat metabolism, ketones are the signal that your liver is now burning energy from fat, not sugar. The liver creates three different types of ketones: acetone, measured in the breath; acetoacetate, measured in the urine; and beta hydroxybutyrate (BHB), measured in the blood. I suggest testing blood ketone measurements for BHB; the optimal range is 0.5–3.0 mmol/L (millimoles per liter).

Ketosis: A metabolic process that occurs when your body doesn't have enough carbohydrates to burn for energy. When you restrict carbohydrates in your diet, you lower the hormone insulin, which allows for fat-burning. You can enter ketosis the preferred way, endogenously (from within) by burning fat for fuel, or exogenously (from outside) from exogenous ketones.

Metabolic flexibility: Being metabolically flexible enough to switch between burning sugar (glucose) and burning fat (ketones) without any problems.

Mitochondria: Mitochondria are membrane-bound cell organelles (mitochondrion, singular) that generate most of the chemical energy needed to power the cell's biochemical reactions. Chemical energy produced by the mitochondria is stored in a small molecule called adenosine triphosphate (ATP). Mitochondria contain their own small chromosomes. Mitochondria are also called the powerhouse of the cell.

mTOR: This stands for "mechanistic target of rapamycin." A cellular signaling pathway that gets triggered when amino acids and insulin levels within the cell increase, which usually happens in the fed state. It stimulates anabolic growth and runs counter to autophagy, which is more catabolic in repair. Once stimulated, the mTOR pathway will promote cellular growth.

Stored sugar: The amount of glucose that is stored in tissues like the liver, fat, brain, muscle, and eyes.

Sugar burner: An energy system that burns fuel from the foods you eat. This energy system runs on the glucose created from food, primarily from carbohydrates.

Water fasting: A fast that involves drinking only water. This means a period (usually more than 16 hours) without food, only water.

ENDNOTES

Introduction

1. Hales et al., "Prevalence of Obesity and Severe Obesity Among Adults: United States, 2017–2018," *NCHS Data Brief*, no. 360 (February 2020). https://www.cdc.gov/nchs/data/databriefs/db360-h.pdf.

2. Fryar et al., "Prevalence of Overweight, Obesity, and Severe Obesity Among Adults Aged 20 and Over: United States, 1960–1962 through 2017–2018," *NCHS Health E-Stats* (December 2020). https://www.cdc.gov/nchs/data/hestat/obesity-adult-17-18/overweight-obesity-adults-H.pdf.

3. Harvard T.H. Chan School of Public Health, "Close to Half of U.S. Population Projected to Have Obesity by 2030," press release, December 18, 2019, https://www.hsph.harvard.edu/news/press-releases/half-of-us-to-have-obesity-by-2030/.

4. UNC Gillings School of Global Public Heath, "Only 12 Percent of American Adults Are Metabolically Healthy, Carolina Study Finds," press release, November 28, 2018, https://www.unc.edu/posts/2018/11/28/only-12-percent-of-american-adults-are-metabolically-healthy-carolina-study-finds/.

5. O'Hearn et al., "Trends and Disparities in Cardiometabolic Health Among U.S. Adults, 1999–2018," *Journal of the American College of Cardiology* 80, no. 2 (2022), 138–151. https://doi.org/10.1016/j.jacc.2022.04.046.

6. Loprinzi et al., "Healthy Lifestyle Characteristics and Their Joint Association with Cardiovascular Disease Biomarkers in US Adults," *Mayo Clinic Proceedings* 91, no. 4 (April 2016), 432–442, https://www.mayoclinicproceedings.org/article/S0025-6196(16)00043-4/abstract.

7. Jennifer Karas Montez, "Policy Polarization and Death in the United States," *Temple Law Review* 92, no. 4 (2020), 889–916. https://www.ncbi.nlm.nih.gov/pmc/articles/PMC8442849.

8. P. Boersma, L. I. Black, and B. W. Ward, "Prevalence of Multiple Chronic Conditions Among US Adults, 2018," *Preventing Chronic Disease* 17, no. 200130 (2020). http://dx.doi.org/10.5888/pcd17.200130.

9. "Health Rankings," American Public Health Association, accessed November 25, 2024, https://www.apha.org/topics-and-issues/health-rankings.

10. "Cancer Prevalence: How Many People Have Cancer," American Cancer Society, last modified January 19, 2023, https://www.cancer.org/cancer/survivorship/cancer-prevalence.html.

11. "About Diabetes," Diabetes Caucus, accessed November 25, 2024, https://diabetescaucus-degette.house.gov/facts-and-figures.

12. "National Diabetes Statistics Report," U.S. Centers for Disease Control and Prevention, May 15, 2024, https://www.cdc.gov/diabetes/php/data-research/index.html

13. "About Diabetes," Diabetes Caucus, accessed November 25, 2024, https://diabetescaucus-degette.house.gov/facts-and-figures.

14. Goldenberg et al., "Efficacy and Safety of Low and Very Low Carbohydrate Diets for Type 2 Diabetes Remission: Systematic Review and Meta-Analysis of Published and Unpublished Randomized Trial Data," *BMJ* 372 (2021): m4743. https://doi.org/10.1136/bmj.m4743.

15. Hallberg et al., "Effectiveness and Safety of a Novel Care Model for the Management of Type 2 Diabetes at 1 Year: An Open-Label, Non-Randomized, Controlled Study," *Diabetes Therapy* 9 (2018): 583–612. https://doi.org/10.1007/s13300-018-0373-9.

16. Athinarayanan et al., "Long-Term Effects of a Novel Continuous Remote Care Intervention Including Nutritional Ketosis for the Management of Type 2 Diabetes: A 2-Year Non-randomized Clinical Trial," *Frontiers in Endocrinology* 10, (2019): 348. https://doi.org/10.3389/fendo.2019.00348.

Chapter 1

1. Eppendorf, "How Many Cells Are in Your Body? Probably More Than You Think!" *Beyond Science* (blog), December 4, 2017, https://www.eppendorf.com/us-en/beyond-science/health-medicine/how-many-cells-are-in-your-body-probably-more-than-you-think.

2. O'Hearn et al., "Trends and Disparities in Cardiometabolic Health Among U.S. Adults, 1999-2018," *Journal of the American College of Cardiology* 80, no. 2 (2022): 138–151. https://doi.org/10.1016/j.jacc.2022.04.046.

3. Bruce H. Lipton, "Brains versus Gonads," *Bruce H. Lipton, PhD* (blog), February 8, 2012, https://www.brucelipton.com/brain-versus-gonads/.

4. Bruce H. Lipton, "Insight into Cellular Consciousness," *Bruce H. Lipton, PhD* (blog), last modified April 22, 2024, https://www.brucelipton.com/insight-cellular-consciousness/.

5. Heidi Godman, "Lessons from *The Biggest Loser*," *Harvard Health Publishing* (blog), January 24, 2018, https://www.health.harvard.edu/diet-and-weight-loss/lessons-from-the-biggest-loser.

6. Vasanti S. Malik and Frank B. Hu, "Sweeteners and Risk of Obesity and Type 2 Diabetes: The Role of Sugar-Sweetened Beverages," *Current Diabetes Reports* 12 (January 2012): 195–203. https://doi.org/10.1007/s11892-012-0259-6.

7. Michael Napolitano and Mihai Covasa, "Microbiota Transplant in the Treatment of Obesity and Diabetes: Current and Future Perspectives," *Frontiers in Microbiology* 11 (2020), https://doi.org/10.3389/fmicb.2020.590370.

8. Digestive Disease Week, "First Randomized Controlled Trial of FMT for Obesity Shows Potential Progress," *Medical X Press*, May 9, 2019, https://medicalxpress.com/news/2019-05-randomized-trial-fmt-obesity-potential.html.

9. Hartford Healthcare, "Stool as a Weight-Loss Tool? The Strange-But-True Fecal Transplant Possibilities," *Hartford Healthcare* (blog), September 19, 2019, https://hartfordhealthcare.org/about-us/news-press/news-detail?articleid=22421&publicId=395.

10. Ori Hofmekler, *The Anti-Estrogenic Diet* (Berkeley, CA: North Atlantic Books, 2007), 110.

11. Ahmed et al., "Impact of Intermittent Fasting on Human Health: An Extended Review of Metabolic Cascades." *International Journal of Food Properties* 21, no. 1 (2018): 2700–2713. https://doi.org/10.1080/10942912.2018.1560312.

12. Solimanik et al., "Prolonged Fasting Outperforms Short-Term Fasting in Terms of Glucose Tolerance and Insulin Release: A Randomised Controlled Trial," *British Journal of Nutrition* 130, no. 9 (2023): 1500–1509. https://doi.org/10.1017/S0007114523000557.

Chapter 2

1. "Hormesis," Wikipedia, accessed February 3, 2025, https://en.wikipedia.org/wiki/Hormesis.

2. Chris Opfer and Allison Troutner, "Does Your Body Really Replace Itself Every Seven Years?" *How Stuff Works*, last modified September 22, 2022, https://science.howstuffworks.com/life/cellular-microscopic/does-body-really-replace-seven-years.htm.

3. Thibault et al., "Crosstalk Between Senescent Bone Cells and the Bone Tissue Microenvironment Influences Bone Fragility During Chronological Age and in Diabetes," *Frontiers in Physiology* 13 (2022). https://doi.org/10.3389/fphys.2022.812157.

4. Bussian et al., "Clearance of Senescent Glial Cells Prevents Tau-Dependent Pathology and Cognitive Decline," *Nature* 562 (2018): 578–582. https://doi.org/10.1038/s41586-018-0543-y.

5. National Institute on Aging, "Senescent Brain Cells May Contribute to Alzheimer's Disease," *Research Highlights* (blog), May 26, 2022, https://www.nia.nih.gov/news/senescent-brain-cells-may-contribute-alzheimers-disease.

6. Mayo Clinic Staff, "Health and Zombie Cells in Aging," Mayo Clinic (blog), December 1, 2023, https://newsnetwork.mayoclinic.org/discussion/health-and-zombie-cells-in-aging/.

7. Giarmarco et al., "Daily Mitochondrial Dynamics in Cone Photoreceptors," *Proceedings of the National Academy of Sciences of the United States of America* 117, no. 46 (2020): 28816–28827. https://doi.org/10.1073/pnas.2007827117.

8. Robert K. Naviaux, "Metabolic Features of the Cell Danger Response," *Mitochondrion* 16 (2014): 7–17. https://doi.org/10.1016/j.mito.2013.08.006.

9. Christiakov et al., "Mitochondrial Aging and Age-Related Dysfunction of Mitochondria," *BioMed Research International* (2014). https://pmc.ncbi.nlm.nih.gov/articles/PMC4003832/.

10. C. Özkul, M. Yalınay, and T. Karakan, T, "Islamic Fasting Leads to an Increased Abundance of Akkermansia Muciniphila and Bacteroides Fragilis Group: A Preliminary Study on Intermittent Fasting," *The Turkish Journal of Gastroenterology* 30, no. 12 (2019): 1030–1035. https://doi.org/10.5152/tjg.2019.19185.

11. Nadeem Khan et al., "Intermittent Fasting Positively Modulates Human Gut Microbial Diversity and Ameliorates Blood Lipid Profile," *Frontiers in Microbiology* 13 (2022). https://doi.org/10.3389/fmicb.2022.922727.

12. Weir et al., "Heart Disease and Cancer Deaths—Trends and Projections in the United States, 1969–2020," *CME Activity* 13 (November 2016). http://dx.doi.org/10.5888/pcd13.160211.

13. Sara Novak, "Type 2 Diabetes Linked with an Increased Risk of Dying from Cancer," *NewScientist*, January 24, 2023, https://www.newscientist.com/article/2356182-type-2-diabetes-linked-with-an-increased-risk-of-dying-from-cancer/.

14. Yadira Galindo, "When—Not What—Obese Mice Ate Reduced Breast Cancer Risk," *UC San Diego Today*, January 25, 2021, https://today.ucsd.edu/story/when-not-what-obese-mice-ate-reduced-breast-cancer-risk.

15. Manasi et al., "Time-Restricted Feeding Normalizes Hyperinsulinemia to Inhibit Breast Cancer in Obese Postmenopausal Mouse Models," *Nature Communications* 12, no. 1 (2021): 565. https://doi.org/10.1038/s41467-020-20743-7.

16. Bruce H. Lipton, "THINK Beyond Your Genes," *Bruce H. Lipton, PhD* (blog), November, 26, 2018, https://www.brucelipton.com/think-beyond-your-genes-november-2018/.

17. N. N. Dasanayaka, N. D. Sirisena, and N. Samaranayake, "The Effects of Mediation on Length of Telomeres in Healthy Individuals: A Systemic Review," *Systemic Reviews* 10, no. 151 (2021). https://doi.org/10.1186/s13643-021-01699-1.

18. Pennington Biomedical Research Center, "Metabolism Changes with Age, Just Not When You Might Think," *ScienceDaily*, August 12, 2021, https://www.sciencedaily.com/releases/2021/08/210812145028.htm?.

Chapter 3

1. Heald et al., "Estimating Life Years Lost to Diabetes: Outcomes from Analysis of National Diabetes Audit and Office of National Statistics Data," *Cardiovascular Endocrinology & Metabolism* 9, no. 4 (2020): 183–185. https://doi.org/10.1097/XCE.0000000000000210.

2. Tabák et al., "Trajectories of Glycaemia, Insulin Sensitivity, and Insulin Secretion Before Diagnosis of Type 2 Diabetes: An Analysis from the Whitehall II Study," *The Lancet* 373, no. 9682 (2009): 2215–2221.

3. Nazia Karsan and Peter J. Goadsby, "Migraine Is More Than Just Headache: Is the Link to Chronic Fatigue and Mood Disorders Simply Due to Shared Biological Systems?" *Frontiers in Human Neuroscience* 15 (2021). https://doi.org/10.3389/fnhum.2021.646692.

4. S. E. Lakhan and A. Kirchgessner, "Gut Inflammation in Chronic Fatigue Syndrome," *Nutrition and Metabolism* 7, no. 79 (2010). https://doi.org/10.1186/1743-7075-7-79.

5. Pedro Rojas-Morales, José Pedraza-Chaverri, and Edilia Tapia, "Ketone Bodies, Stress Response, and Redox Homeostasis," *Redox Biology* 29 (2020). https://doi.org/10.1016/j.redox.2019.101395.

6. Roberts et al., "A Ketogenic Diet Extends Longevity and Healthspan in Adult Mice," *Cell Metabolism* 26, no. 3 (2017): 539–546.e5. https://doi.org/10.1016/j.cmet.2017.08.005.

7. Newman et al., "Ketogenic Diet Reduces Midlife Mortality and Improves Memory in Aging Mice," *Cell Metabolism* 26, no 3 (2017): 547–557.e8. https://doi.org/10.1016/j.cmet.2017.08.004.

8. Shimazu et al., "Suppression of Oxidative Stress by β-hydroxybutyrate, an Endogenous Histone Deacetylase Inhibitor," *Science* 339, no. 6116 (2013): 211–214. https://doi.org/10.1126/science.1227166.

9. S. M. de la Monte and J. R. Wands, "Alzheimer's Disease Is Type 3 Diabetes—Evidence Reviewed," *Journal of Diabetes Science and Technology* 2, no. 6 (2008): 1101–1113. https://doi.org/10.1177/193229680800200619.

10. Jensen et al., "Effects of Ketone Bodies on Brain Metabolism and Function in Neurodegenerative Diseases," *International Journal of Molecular Sciences* 21, no. 22 (2020): 8767. https://doi.org/10.3390/ijms21228767.

11. H. Hersant and G. Grossberg, "The Ketogenic Diet and Alzheimer's Disease," *Journal of Nutrition, Health & Aging* 26, no. 6 (2022): 606–614. https://doi.org/10.1007/s12603-022-1807-7.

12. E. Ozan, V. A. Chouinard, and C. M. Palmer, "The Ketogenic Diet as a Treatment for Mood Disorders," *Current Treatment Options in Psychiatry* 11 (2024): 163–176. https://doi.org/10.1007/s40501-024-00322-z.

13. Kelsie Smith Hayduk, "Can Ketones Enhance Cognitive Function and Protect Brain Networks?" *University of Rochester Medical Center Newsroom*, May 31, 2024, https://www.urmc.rochester.edu/news/publications/neuroscience/can-ketones-enhance-cognitive-function-and-protect-brain-networks.

14. The Physiological Society, "Ketone Supplement Might Be a Novel Therapeutic for Boosting Brain Function in Obesity," *ScienceDaily*, October 5, 2021, https://www.sciencedaily.com/releases/2021/10/211005101908.htm.

15. Fisher Center for Alzheimer's Research Foundation, "Nearly 14 Million Americans Will Have Alzheimer's Disease by 2060," December 5, 2060, https://www.alzinfo.org/articles/research/nearly-14-million-americans-will-have-alzheimers-disease-by-2060/.

16. M. V. Liberti and J. W. Locasale, "The Warburg Effect: How Does It Benefit Cancer Cells?" *Trends in Biochemical Sciences* 41, no. 3 (2016): 211–218. https://doi.org/10.1016/j.tibs.2015.12.001.

17. J. Tan-Shalaby, "Ketogenic Diets and Cancer: Emerging Evidence," *Federal Practitioner* 34, Suppl. 1 (2017): 37S–42S. https://pubmed.ncbi.nlm.nih.gov/30766299/.

18. Tan-Shalaby, "Ketogenic Diets and Cancer." *Federal Practitioner* 34, Suppl. 1 (2017): 37S–42S. https://pubmed.ncbi.nlm.nih.gov/30766299/.

Chapter 4

1. Michele Majidi, "Pharmaceutical Industry TV Advertising Spending in the United States from 2016 to 2020." Statista, December 20, 2023. https://www.statista.com/statistics/953104/pharma-industry-tv-ad-spend-us/.

2. Harvard Health Publishing, "Do Not Get Sold on Drug Advertising," *Harvard Health Publishing* (blog), February 14, 2017, https://www.health.harvard.edu/medications/do-not-get-sold-on-drug-advertising.

3. Anthony E. Gallo, "Food Advertising in the United States," in *America's Eating Habits: Changes and Consequences*, Elizabeth Frazão, ed., (Washington, DC: U.S. Department of Agriculture, 1999), https://ers.usda.gov/sites/default/files/_laserfiche/publications/42215/5838_aib750i_1_.pdf

4. The Commonwealth Fund, "U.S. Ranks Last Among Seven Countries on Health System Performance Measures," newsletter, accessed November 26, 2024, https://www.commonwealthfund.org/publications/newsletter-article/us-ranks-last-among-seven-countries-health-system-performance.

5. R. Petersen, L. Pan, and H. M. Blanck, "Racial and Ethnic Disparities in Adult Obesity in the United States: CDC's Tracking to Inform State and Local Action," *Preventing Chronic Disease* 16 (2019). http://dx.doi.org/10.5888/pcd16.180579.

6. Parker et al., "Economic Costs of Diabetes in the U.S. in 2022," *Diabetes Care* 47, no. 1 (2024): 26–43. https://doi.org/10.2337/dci23-0085.

7. Vitale et al., "Ultra-Processed Foods and Human Health: A Systematic Review and Meta-Analysis of Prospective Cohort Studies," *Advances in Nutrition* 15, no. 1 (2024). https://doi.org/10.1016/j.advnut.2023.09.009.

8. Kashmira Gander, "Doritos Roulette: School Warns Parents Not to Give Children Crisps After Pupil Left Struggling to Breathe," *The Independent*, July 17, 2015, https://www.independent.co.uk/lifestyle/health-and-families/health-news/doritos-roulette-school-warns-parents-not-to-give-children-crisps-after-pupil-was-left-struggling-to-breathe-10393965.html.

9. N. M. Avena, P. Rada, and B. G. Hoebel, "Evidence for Sugar Addiction: Behavioral and Neurochemical Effects of Intermittent, Excessive Sugar Intake," *Neuroscience and Biobehavioral Reviews* 32, no. 1 (2008): 20–39. https://doi.org/10.1016/j.neubiorev.2007.04.019.

10. Diabetes Research & Wellness Foundation, "Most People in the UK Consume 3 Times the Advised Daily Sugar Intake," news release, March 28, 2018, https://www.drwf.org.uk/news-and-events/news/report-on-diet-finds-most-people-in-the-uk-are-consuming-almost-3-times-the-recommended-daily-sugar-intake/.

11. Alessio Fasano, "All Disease Begins in the (Leaky) Gut: Role of Zonulin-Mediated Gut Permeability in the Pathogenesis of Some Chronic Inflammatory Diseases," *F1000Research* 9 (2020): https://doi.org/10.12688/f1000research.20510.1.

Chapter 5

1. Environmental Working Group, "Body Burdens: The Pollution in Newborns," *EWG Research* (blog), July 14, 2005, https://www.ewg.org/research/body-burden-pollution-newborns.

2. Anand et al., "Cancer Is a Preventable Disease That Requires Major Lifestyle Changes," *Pharmaceutical Research* 25 (2008): 2097–2116. https://doi.org/10.1007/s11095-008-9661-9.

3. Minnesota Pollution Control Agency, "BPA and BPS in Thermal Paper," *Business with Us* (blog), accessed November 26, 2024, https://www.pca.state.mn.us/business-with-us/bpa-and-bps-in-thermal-paper.

4. The University of Newcastle, Australia, "Plastic Ingestion by People Could Be Equating to a Credit Card a Week," *University News* (blog), June 12, 2019, https://www.newcastle.edu.au/newsroom/featured/plastic-ingestion-by-people-could-be-equating-to-a-credit-card-a-week.

5. Marfella et al., "Microplastics and Nanoplastics in Atheromas and Cardiovascular Events," *New England Journal of Medicine* 390, no. 10 (March 2024): 900–910. https://doi.org/10.1056/NEJMoa2309822.

6. UniCamillus, "Obesity Alarm in Italy: 12% of the Italian Population Is Obese (Osservasalute Report)," news release, June 23, 2024, https://www.unicamillus.org/obesity-alarm-in-italy-12-of-the-italian-population-is-obese/.

7. Istat, "Diabetes in Italy," press release, July 24, 2017, https://www.istat.it/en/press-release/diabetes-in-italy-years-2000-2016.

8. Health Data Overview for the Republic of Italy," World Health Organization Data, accessed November 26, 2024, https://data.who.int/countries/380.

9. "Life Expectancy," National Center for Health Statistics, October 25, 2024, https://www.cdc.gov/nchs/fastats/life-expectancy.htm.

10. Pesticide Action Network, "Italy Places Important Restrictions on the Use of Glyphosate," press release, August 24, 2016, https://www.pan-europe.info/press-releases/2016/08/italy-places-important-restrictions-use-glyphosate.

11. Tadeu de Araújo-Ramos et al., "Controversies on Endocrine and Reproductive Effects of Glyphosate and Glyphosate-Based Herbicides: A Mini-Review," *Frontiers in Endocrinology* 12 (2021). https://doi.org/10.3389/fendo.2021.627210.

12. A. Samsel and S. Seneff, "Glyphosate, Pathways to Modern Diseases III: Manganese, Neurological Diseases, and Associated Pathologies," *Surgical Neurology International* 6, no. 45 (2015). https://doi.org/10.4103/2152-7806.153876.

13. Feng-chih Chang, Matt F. Simcik, and Paul D. Capel, "Occurrence and Fate of the Herbicide Glyphosate and Its Degradate Aminomethylphosphonic Acid in the Atmosphere," *Environmental Toxicology and Chemistry* 30, no. 3 (2011): 548–555. https://doi.org/10.1002/etc.431.

14. J. Y. Jeon, K. H. Ha, and D. J. Kim, "New Risk Factors for Obesity and Diabetes: Environmental Chemicals," *Journal of Diabetes Investigation* 6, no. 2 (2015): 109–111. https://doi.org/10.1111/jdi.12318.

15. W. Holtcamp, "Obesogens: An Environmental Link to Obesity," *Environmental Health Perspectives* 120, no. 2 (2012): a62–a68. https://doi.org/10.1289/ehp.120-a62.

16. "Common EDCs and Where They Are Found," Endocrine Society, accessed November 26, 2024, https://www.endocrine.org/topics/edc/what-edcs-are/common-edcs.

17. Philippa D. Darbre, "Endocrine Disruptors and Obesity," *Current Obesity Reports* 6 (2017): 18–27. https://doi.org/10.1007/s13679-017-0240-4.

18. W. Holtcamp, "Obesogens: An Environmental Link to Obesity," *Environmental Health Perspectives* 120, no. 2 (2012): a62–a68. https://doi.org/10.1289/ehp.120-a62.

19. Philippa D. Darbre, "Endocrine Disruptors and Obesity," *Current Obesity Reports* 6 (2017): 18–27. https://doi.org/10.1007/s13679-017-0240-4.

Chapter 6

1. Laura Smith, "53 Sleep Statistics: What Percentage of the Population Is Sleep Deprived?" *The Good Body* (blog), November 23, 2022, https://www.thegoodbody.com/sleep-statistics/.

2. Nina Julia, "Sleep Statistics: Facts & Latest Data in America (2024 Update)," CFAH, last updated January 11, 2024. https://cfah.org/sleep-statistics/.

3. Julia Forbes, "54 Sleep Statistics and Trends for 2024," *Sleep Advisor*, September 3, 2024, https://www.sleepadvisor.org/sleep-statistics/.

4. Donya Currie, ed., "Sleep Statistics and Facts," *National Council on Aging* (blog), March 7, 2024, https://www.ncoa.org/adviser/sleep/sleep-statistics/.

5. Eric Suni and Kimberly Truong, "100+ Sleep Statistics," *Sleep Foundation* (blog), September 26, 2023, https://www.sleepfoundation.org/how-sleep-works/sleep-facts-statistics.

6. Nina Julia, "Sleep Statistics: Facts & Latest Data in America (2024 Update)," CFAH, last updated January 11, 2024. https://cfah.org/sleep-statistics/.

7. Suni and Truong, "100+ Sleep Statistics." *Sleep Foundation* (blog), September 26, 2023, https://www.sleepfoundation.org/how-sleep-works/sleep-facts-statistics.

8. Donya Currie, ed., "Sleep Statistics and Facts." *National Council on Aging* (blog), March 7, 2024, https://www.ncoa.org/adviser/sleep/sleep-statistics/.

9. Institute of Medicine (US) Committee on Sleep Medicine and Research, *Sleep Disorders and Sleep Deprivation: An Unmet Public Health Problem*, edited by H. R. Colten and B. M. Altevogt (Washington, D.C.: National Academies Press, 2006), chap. 4, https://www.ncbi.nlm.nih.gov/books/NBK19958/.

10. Van Cauter et al., "Metabolic Consequences of Sleep and Sleep Loss," *Sleep Medicine* 9, Suppl. (2008): S23–S28. https://doi.org/10.1016/S1389-9457(08)70013-3.

11. American College of Physicians, "Short-Term Sleep Deprivation Significantly Decreases Insulin Sensitivity in Fat Cells," *ACP Newsroom*, October 15, 2012, https://www.acponline.org/acp-newsroom/short-term-sleep-deprivation-significantly-decreases-insulin-sensitivity-in-fat-cells.

12. Roo Killick, Siobhan Banks, and Peter Y. Liu, "Implications of Sleep Restriction and Recovery on Metabolic Outcomes," *The Journal of Clinical Endocrinology & Metabolism* 97, no. 11 (November 2012): 3876–3890. https://doi.org/10.1210/jc.2012-1845.

13. University of Chicago Medical Center, "Even Your Fat Cells Need Sleep, According to New Research," *ScienceDaily*, October 15, 2012, www.sciencedaily.com/releases/2012/10/121015170822.htm.

14. Buxton et al., "Sleep Restriction for 1 Week Reduces Insulin Sensitivity in Healthy Men," *Diabetes* 59, no. 1 (June 2010): 2126–2133. https://doi.org/10.2337/db09-0699.

15. Zamani-Alavijeh et al., "The Effectiveness of Stress Management Training on Blood Glucose Control in Patients with Type 2 Diabetes," *Diabetology & Metabolic Syndrome* 10, no. 39 (2018). https://doi.org/10.1186/s13098-018-0342-5.

16. K. Spiegel, R. Leproult, and E. Van Cauter, "Impact of Sleep Debt on Metabolic and Endocrine Function," *Lancet* 354, no. 9188 (1999): 1435–1439. https://doi.org/10.1016/S0140-6736(99)01376-8.

17. Ayas et al., "A Prospective Study of Self-Reported Sleep Duration and Incident Diabetes in Women," *Diabetes Care* 26, no. 2 (2003): 380–384. https://doi.org/10.2337/diacare.26.2.380.

18. Axelsson et al., "Sleepiness as Motivation: A Potential Mechanism for How Sleep Deprivation Affects Behavior," *Sleep* 43, no. 6 (June 2020): zsz291. https://doi.org/10.1093/sleep/zsz291.

19. World Health Organization, "IARC Monographs Volume 124: Night Shift Work," *IARC News*, June 2, 2020, https://www.iarc.who.int/news-events/iarc-monographs-volume-124-night-shift-work/.

20. Windred et al., "Sleep Regularity Is a Stronger Predictor of Mortality Risk Than Sleep Duration: A Prospective Cohort Study," *Sleep* 47, no. 1 (January 2024): zsad253. https://doi.org/10.1093/sleep/zsad253.

21. Salk Institute, "Time-Restricted Eating Reshapes Gene Expression throughout the Body," *Salk News*, press release, January 3, 2023, https://www.salk.edu/news-release/time-restricted-eating-reshapes-gene-expression-throughout-the-body.

22. RNZ, "Eating Times Essential to Healthy Diet and Nutrition—Dr. Satchin Panda," *RNZ Health* (blog), August 7, 2018, https://www.rnz.co.nz/national/programmes/afternoons/audio/2018657024/eating-times-essential-to-healthy-diet-and-nutrition-dr-satchin-panda.

23. Salk Institute, "Eating in 10-hour Window Can Override Disease-Causing Genetic Defects, Nurture Health," *Salk News*, press release, August 30, 2018, https://www.salk.edu/news-release/eating-in-10-hour-window-can-override-disease-causing-genetic-defects-nurture-health.

24. Salk Institute, "Clinical Study Finds Eating within a 10-Hour Window May Help Stave Off Diabetes, Heart Disease," *Salk News*, press release, December 5, 2019, https://www.salk.edu/news-release/clinical-study-finds-eating-within-10-hour-window-may-help-stave-off-diabetes-heart-disease.

25. Salk Institute, "Satchidananda Panda, PhD," (faculty profile), accessed November 27, 2024, https://www.salk.edu/scientist/satchidananda-panda.

26. Salk Institute, "Time-restricted Eating Reshapes Gene Expression throughout the Body," *Salk News*, press release, January 3, 2023, https://www.salk.edu/news-release/time-restricted-eating-reshapes-gene-expression-throughout-the-body.

27. Salk Institute, "Clinical Study Finds Eating within a 10-Hour Window May Help Stave Off Diabetes, Heart Disease," *Salk News*, press release, December 5, 2019, https://www.salk.edu/news-release/clinical-study-finds-eating-within-10-hour-window-may-help-stave-off-diabetes-heart-disease.

Chapter 7

1. Mary K. Enig, Ph.D., "Fat and Cholesterol in Human Milk," *Weston A. Price Foundation* (blog), December 31, 2001, https://www.westonaprice.org/health-topics/fat-and-cholesterol-in-human-milk.

2. Khalid et al., "Effects of Ketogenic Diet on Reproductive Hormones in Women with Polycystic Ovary Syndrome," *Journal of the Endocrine Society* 7, no. 10 (October 2023): bvad112. https://doi.org/10.1210/jendso/bvad112.

3. Johns Hopkins Medicine, "Keto Diet Therapy Recommendations Set for Adults with Epilepsy, Other Neurologic Diseases," *Johns Hopkins Medicine Newsroom*, November 24, 2020, https://clinicalconnection.hopkinsmedicine.org/news/keto-diet-therapy-recommendations-set-for-adults-with-epilepsy-other-neurologic-diseases.

4. Rusek et al., "Ketogenic Diet in Alzheimer's Disease," *International Journal of Molecular Sciences* 20, no. 16 (2019): 3892. https://doi.org/10.3390/ijms20163892.

5. Shahpasand et al., "Therapeutic Potential of the Ketogenic Diet: A Metabolic Switch with Implications for Neurological Disorders, the Gut-Brain Axis, and Cardiovascular Diseases," *Journal of Nutritional Biochemistry* 132, no. 109693 (2024). https://doi.org/10.1016/j.jnutbio.2024.109693.

6. Eugene Reznick, "A Review of the Ketogenic Diet in the Treatment of Autism Spectrum Disorder," Ph.D. diss., Loma Linda University, 2024, https://scholarsrepository.llu.edu/etd/1713.

7. M. Grootveld, "Evidence-Based Challenges to the Continued Recommendation and Use of Peroxidatively-Susceptible Polyunsaturated Fatty Acid-Rich Culinary Oils for High-Temperature Frying Practises: Experimental Revelations Focused on Toxic Aldehydic Lipid Oxidation Products," *Frontiers in Nutrition* 8, no. 711640 (2022). https://doi.org/10.3389/fnut.2021.711640.

8. "List of 100 Top Selling Grocery Items 2025 & Tips," *BusinessNes,* updated January 8, 2025, https://businessnes.com/list-of-top-selling-grocery-items-and-tips/.

9. Ekaterina Pesheva, "Diet, Gut Microbes, and Immunity," *Harvard Medical School News & Research* (blog), November 16, 2021, https://hms.harvard.edu/news/diet-gut-microbes-immunity

10. Melina Roberts, "Five Connections between Bile Flow and Thyroid Function," Advanced Naturopathic Medical Centre, accessed November 27, 2024, https://advancednaturopathic.com/bile-thyroid-connection.

11. J. Laukkarinen, J. Sand, and I. Nordback, "The Underlying Mechanisms: How Hypothyroidism Affects the Formation of Common Bile Duct Stones," *HPB Surgery*, no. 102825 (2012). https://doi.org/10.1155/2012/102825.

12. Nazia Karsan and Peter J. Goadsby, "Migraine Is More Than Just Headache: Is the Link to Chronic Fatigue and Mood Disorders Simply Due to Shared Biological Systems?" *Frontiers in Human Neuroscience* 15 (2021). https://doi.org/10.3389/fnhum.2021.646692.

13. Ravindran et al., "Migraine Headaches in Chronic Fatigue Syndrome (CFS): Comparison of Two Prospective Cross-Sectional Studies," *BMC Neurology* 11, no. 30 (2011). https://doi.org/10.1186/1471-2377-11-30.

14. S. E. Lakhan and A. Kirchgessner, "Gut Inflammation in Chronic Fatigue Syndrome," *Nutrition & Metabolism* 7, no. 79 (2010). https://doi.org/10.1186/1743-7075-7-79.

15. American Association for the Advancement of Science, "Coffee Is Number One Source of Antioxidants," news release, August 28, 2005, https://www.eurekalert.org/news-releases/560866.

16. Hassan Baky et al., "Interactions between Dietary Flavonoids and the Gut Microbiome: A Comprehensive Review," *British Journal of Nutrition* 128, no. 4 (2022): 577–591. https://doi.org/10.1017/S0007114521003627.

Chapter 8

1. American Heart Association, "More Than 100 Million Americans Have High Blood Pressure, AHA Says," news release, January 31, 2018, https://www.heart.org/en/news/2018/07/18/more-than-100-million-americans-have-high-blood-pressure-aha-says.

2. Jaws Podiatry, "How High Blood Pressure Affects Your Feet," *Jaws Podiatry* (blog), accessed November 27, 2024, https://www.jawspodiatry.com/how-high-blood-pressure-affects-your-feet.

3. Benedict et al., *A Study of Prolonged Fasting* (Washington, D.C.: Carnegie Institution of Washington, 1915), https://archive.org/details/cu31924003162959.

4. Goldhamer et al., "Medically Supervised Water-Only Fasting in the Treatment of Hypertension," *Journal of Manipulative and Physiological Therapeutics* 24, no. 5 (June 2001), https://www.truenorthhealthfoundation.org/sites/default/files/docs/fasting-database-article/Goldhamer%20et%20al_2001_Medically%20Supervised%20Water-only%20Fasting%20in%20the%20Treatment%20of%20Hypertension.pdf.

5. Anne Tafton, "Fasting Boosts Stem Cells' Regenerative Capacity," *MIT News* (blog), May 3, 2018, https://news.mit.edu/2018/fasting-boosts-stem-cells-regenerative-capacity-0503.

6. Mihaylova et al., "Fasting Activates Fatty Acid Oxidation to Enhance Intestinal Stem Cell Function during Homeostasis and Aging," *Cell Stem Cell* 22 (2018): 769–778. https://dspace.mit.edu/handle/1721.1/124714.

7. Godínez-Victoria et al., "Intermittent Fasting Promotes Bacterial Clearance and Intestinal IgA Production in *Salmonella typhimurium*-Infected Mice," *Scandinavian Journal of Immunology* 79, no. 5 (2014): 283–345. https://onlinelibrary.wiley.com/doi/epdf/10.1111/sji.12163.

8. Li et al., "Intermittent Fasting Promotes White Adipose Browning and Decreases Obesity by Shaping the Gut Microbiota," *Cell Metabolism* 26, no. 4 (2017): 672–685.e4. https://doi.org/10.1016/j.cmet.2017.08.019.

9. Khan et al., "Intermittent Fasting Positively Modulates Human Gut Microbial Diversity and Ameliorates Blood Lipid Profile," *Frontiers in Microbiology* 13 (2022). https://doi.org/10.3389/fmicb.2022.922727.

10. M. P. Mattson, "Energy Intake, Meal Frequency, and Health: A Neurobiological Perspective," *Annual Review of Nutrition*, 25 (2005): 237–260. https://doi.org/10.1146/annurev.nutr.25.050304.092526.

11. Brian Doctrow, "Calorie Restriction, Immune Function, and Health Span," *NIH Research Matters* (blog), March 1, 2022, https://www.nih.gov/news-events/nih-research-matters/calorie-restriction-immune-function-health-span.

12. Chantal Gil, "The Starvation Experiment," *Duke Psychiatry & Behavioral Services* (blog), May 9, 2023, https://psychiatry.duke.edu/blog/starvation-experiment.

13. Zauner et al., "Resting Energy Expenditure in Short-Term Starvation Is Increased as a Result of an Increase in Serum Norepinephrine," *American Journal of Clinical Nutrition* 71, no. 6 (2000): 1511–1515. https://doi.org/10.1093/ajcn/71.6.1511.

14. Ouellet et al., "Brown Adipose Tissue Oxidative Metabolism Contributes to Energy Expenditure During Acute Cold Exposure in Humans," *Journal of Clinical Investigation* 122, no. 2 (2012): 545–552. https://doi.org/10.1172/JCI60433.

15. Max Bingham, "New Obesity Tool?" *Harvard Medical School News & Research*, April 14, 2001, https://hms.harvard.edu/news/new-obesity-tool.

16. Endocrine Society, "People with Brown Fat May Burn 15 Percent More Calories," press release, April 28, 2020, https://www.endocrine.org/news-and-advocacy/news-room/2020/people-with-brown-fat-may-burn-15-percent-more-calories.

17. Diab et al., "Intermittent Fasting Regulates Metabolic Homeostasis and Improves Cardiovascular Health," *Cell Biochemistry and Biophysics* 82 (2024): 1583–1597. https://doi.org/10.1007/s12013-024-01314-9.

18. Kaylyn Tousignant, "What Science Says About Intermittent Fasting and the Gut Microbiome," *Co-Biome by Microba* report, June 10, 2024, https://www.co-biome.com/education/patient/what-science-says-about-intermittent-fasting-and-the-gut-microbiome.

19. Ducarmon et al., "Long-Term Fasting Remodels Gut Microbial Metabolism and Host Metabolism," *bioRxiv* (preprint) (April 19, 2024), https://doi.org/10.1101/2024.04.19.590209.

Chapter 9

1. Chiavaroli et al., "Effect of Low Glycaemic Index or Load Dietary Patterns on Glycaemic Control and Cardiometabolic Risk Factors in Diabetes: Systematic Review and Meta-Analysis of Randomised Controlled Trials," *BMJ* 374 (2021): 1651. https://doi.org/10.1136/bmj.n1651.

2. L. Nesti, A. Mengozzi, and D. Tricò, "Impact of Nutrient Type and Sequence on Glucose Tolerance: Physiological Insights and Therapeutic Implications," *Frontiers in Endocrinology* 10 (2019): 144. https://doi.org/10.3389/fendo.2019.00144.

3. Laura Williamson, "To Curb High Rates of Heart Disease and Stroke, Experts Urge Prevention and Innovation," American Heart Association news release, January 24, 2024, https://www.heart.org/en/news/2024/01/24/to-curb-high-rates-of-heart-disease-and-stroke-experts-urge-prevention-and-innovation.

4. Dominic Lawson, "Warnings about Blood Pressure? I Take Them with a Pinch of Salt, Says Dominic Lawson," *Daily Mail*, May 29, 2017, https://www.dailymail.co.uk/debate/article-4551028/Blood-pressure-warnings-pinch-salt.html.

5. The Cornucopia Institute, "Apeel and Edible Coatings: Your Questions Answered," Cornucopia News release, updated August 9, 2023, https://www.cornucopia.org/2023/07/apeel-and-edible-coatings-your-questions-answered/.

6. "Study: Hot Dogs May Raise Risk of Childhood Leukemia," *Supermarket News*, June 13, 1994, https://www.supermarketnews.com/grocery-operations/study-hot-dogs-may-raise-risk-of-childhood-leukemia.

7. Amy-Sarah Mitchell, "Do Hot Dogs Cause Cancer? Processed Meat & Colon Cancer," *UVAHealth* (blog), March 3, 2023, https://blog.uvahealth.com/2023/03/02/do-hot-dogs-cause-cancer.

8. Cioffi et al., "Fructose-Rich Diet Affects Mitochondrial DNA Damage and Repair in Rats," *Nutrients* 9, no. 4 (2017): 323. https://doi.org/10.3390/nu9040323.

9. Dornas et al., "Health Implications of High-Fructose Intake and Current Research," *Advances in Nutrition* 6, no. 6 (2015): 729–737. https://doi.org/10.3945/an.114.008144.

10. Jonathan Q. Purnell and Damien A. Fair, "Fructose Ingestion and Cerebral, Metabolic, and Satiety Responses," *JAMA* 309, no. 1 (2013): 85–86. https://doi.org/10.1001/jama.2012.190505.

11. Hieronimus et al., "Effects of Consuming Beverages Sweetened with Fructose, Glucose, High-Fructose Corn Syrup, Sucrose, or Aspartame on OGTT-Derived Indices of Insulin Sensitivity in Young Adults," *Nutrients* 16, no. 1 (2024): 151. https://doi.org/10.3390/nu16010151.

12. Aeberli et al., "Moderate Amounts of Fructose Consumption Impair Insulin Sensitivity in Healthy Young Men: A Randomized Controlled Trial," *Diabetes Care* 36, no. 1 (2013): 150–156. https://doi.org/10.2337/dc12-0540.

13. Jensen et al., "Fructose and Sugar: A Major Mediator of Non-Alcoholic Fatty Liver Disease," *Journal of Hepatology* 68, no. 5 (2018): 1063–1075. https://doi.org/10.1016/j.jhep.2018.01.019.

14. Raatz et al., "Consumption of Honey, Sucrose, and High-Fructose Corn Syrup Produces Similar Metabolic Effects in Glucose-Tolerant and -Intolerant Individuals," *Journal of Nutrition* 145, no. 10 (2015): 2265–2272. https://doi.org/10.3945/jn.115.218016.

15. Stanhope et al., "A Dose-Response Study of Consuming High-Fructose Corn Syrup–Sweetened Beverages on Lipid/Lipoprotein Risk Factors for Cardiovascular Disease in Young Adults," *American Journal of Clinical Nutrition* 101, no. 6 (2015): 1144–1154. https://doi.org/10.3945/ajcn.114.100461.

16. Stanhope et al., "Consumption of Fructose and High Fructose Corn Syrup Increase Postprandial Triglycerides, LDL-Cholesterol, and Apolipoprotein-B in Young Men and Women," *Journal of Clinical Endocrinology & Metabolism* 96, no. 10 (2011): E1596–E1605. https://doi.org/10.1210/jc.2011-1251.

17. Jameel et al., "Acute Effects of Feeding Fructose, Glucose and Sucrose on Blood Lipid Levels and Systemic Inflammation," *Lipids in Health and Disease* 13, no. 195 (2014). https://doi.org/10.1186/1476-511X-13-195.

18. Pett et al., "The Seven Countries Study," *European Heart Journal* 38, no. 42 (2017): 3119–3121. https://doi.org/10.1093/eurheartj/ehx603.

19. John Gordon Harold, "Harold on History | Myocardial Infarction: Evolution in Diagnosis, Care, Prognosis," *Cardiology Magazine*, 2019, https://www.acc.org/Latest-in-Cardiology/Articles/2019/01/07/12/42/Harold-on-History-Myocardial-Infarction-Evolution-in-Diagnosis-Care-Prognosis.

20. J. M. Ketchem, E. J. Bowman, and C. M. Isales, "Male Sex Hormones, Aging, and Inflammation," *Biogerontology* 24 (2023): 1–25. https://doi.org/10.1007/s10522-022-10002-1.

21. Daniel Kelly, "Low Testosterone in Men Associated with an Early Death," *Medical Xpress*, May 15, 2024, https://medicalxpress.com/news/2024-05-testosterone-men-early-death.html.

22. J. M. Ketchem, E. J. Bowman, and C. M. Isales, "Male Sex Hormones, Aging, and Inflammation," *Biogerontology* 24 (2023): 1–25. https://doi.org/10.1007/s10522-022-10002-1.

23. "Protein Leverage Hypothesis," Wikipedia, accessed December 2, 2024, https://en.wikipedia.org/wiki/Protein_leverage_hypothesis.

24. Holt et al., "A Satiety Index of Common Foods," *European Journal of Clinical Nutrition* 49, no. 9 (1995): 675–690. https://researchers.mq.edu.au/en/publications/a-satiety-index-of-common-foods.

Chapter 10

1. "Psycho-Cybernetics," Wikipedia, accessed December 2, 2024, https://en.wikipedia.org/wiki/Psycho-Cybernetics.

2. Joel Arthur Baker, *Paradigms: The Business of Discovering the Future* (New York: HarperBusiness, 1993), https://archive.org/details/paradigmsbusines00bark.

3. Susan Perry, "The Power of the Placebo," BrainFacts.org, May 31, 2012, https://www.brainfacts.org/archives/2012/the-power-of-the-placebo.

4. AP, "'Hysteria' Among Possible Causes of Illness of 125 at Game on Coast," *New York Times*, October 24, 1982, https://www.nytimes.com/1982/10/24/us/hysteria-among-possible-causes-of-illness-of-125-at-game-on-coast.html.

5. Peggy McColl, "Faith Is Powerful," *Proctor Gallagher Institute* (blog), accessed November 27, 2024, https://www.proctorgallagherinstitute.com/38329/faith-is-powerful.

6. Joe Dispenza, "The Power of Gratitude," *Unlimited* (blog), November 25, 2016, https://drjoedispenza.com/blogs/dr-joes-blog/the-power-of-gratitude.

7. Margaret Rhea, "Gratitude," UC Davis Health Wellness News 49 (November 2019), https://health.ucdavis.edu/nursing/academics/studentwellness/pdfs/BIMSON_Newsletter-November_2019.pdf.

8. Picard et al., "A Mitochondrial Health Index Sensitive to Mood and Caregiving Stress," *Biological Psychiatry* 84, no. 1 (2018): 9–17. https://doi.org/10.1016/j.biopsych.2018.01.012.

9. Chen et al., "Gratitude and Mortality Among Older US Female Nurses," *JAMA Psychiatry* 81, no. 10 (2024): 1030–1038. https://doi.org/10.1001/jamapsychiatry.2024.1687.

10. Goodreads, "Quotable Quote," Robert A. Heinlein, accessed January 26, 2025, https://www.goodreads.com/quotes/73503-in-the-absence-of-clearly-defined-goals-we-become-strangely-loyal.

11. A. G. Barnett and A. J. Dobson, "Excess in Cardiovascular Events on Mondays: A Meta-Analysis and Prospective Study," *Journal of Epidemiology and Community Health* 59, no. 2 (2005): 109–114. https://doi.org/10.1136/jech.2003.019489.

12. Pindek et al., "Workdays Are Not Created Equal: Job Satisfaction and Job Stressors Across the Workweek," *Human Relations* 74, no. 9 (2021): 1447–1472. https://doi.org/10.1177/0018726720924444.

13. Maria J. Fitzpatrick and Timothy J. Moore, "The Mortality Effects of Retirement: Evidence from Social Security Eligibility at Age 62," *National Bureau of Economic Research*, Working Paper Series 24127, December 2017, http://www.nber.org/papers/w24127.

14. Pagnini et al., "Ageing as a Mindset: A Study Protocol to Rejuvenate Older Adults with a Counterclockwise Psychological Intervention," *BMJ* 9, no. 7 (2019): e030411. https://doi.org/10.1136/bmjopen-2019-030411.

15. Ellen Langer and Judith Rodin, "The Effects of Choice and Enhanced Personal Responsibility for the Aged: A Field Experiment in an Institutional Setting," *Journal of Personality and Social Psychology* 34, no. 2 (August 1976): 191–198. https://doi.org/10.1037/0022-3514.34.2.191.

16. Benjamin Hardy, "Age Does Not Define You; You Can Be Whoever You Want to Be," *Thought.is*, accessed November 27, 2024, https://thought.is/age-does-not-define-you-you-can-be-whoever-you-want-to-be.

17. Dan Gordon, "Laughing All the Way," *UCLA Magazine*, July 1, 2019, https://newsroom.ucla.edu/magazine/norman-cousins-humor-health-mind-body.

18. Funakubo et al., "Effects of a Laughter Program on Body Weight and Mental Health Among Japanese People with Metabolic Syndrome Risk Factors: A Randomized Controlled Trial," *BMC Geriatrics* 22, no. 361 (2022). https://doi.org/10.1186/s12877-022-03038-y.

19. American Physiological Society, "Laughter Remains Good Medicine," *ScienceDaily*, accessed November 27, 2024, www.sciencedaily.com/releases/2009/04/090417084115.htm.

Chapter 11

1. Watanabe et al., "Coffee Abundant in Chlorogenic Acids Reduces Abdominal Fat in Overweight Adults: A Randomized, Double-Blind, Controlled Trial," *Nutrients* 11, no. 7 (2019): 1617. https://doi.org/10.3390/nu11071617.

2. J. H. O'Keefe, J. J. DiNicolantonio, and C. J. Lavie, "Coffee for Cardioprotection and Longevity," *Progress in Cardiovascular Diseases* 61, no. 1 (2018): 38–42. https://doi.org/10.1016/j.pcad.2018.02.002.

3. Wu et al., "Chlorogenic Acid Protects Against Atherosclerosis in Apoe⁻/⁻ Mice and Promotes Cholesterol Efflux from RAW264.7 Macrophages," *PloS One* 9, no. 9 (2014): e95452. https://doi.org/10.1371/journal.pone.0095452.

4. N. Liang and D. D. Kitts, "Role of Chlorogenic Acids in Controlling Oxidative and Inflammatory Stress Conditions," *Nutrients* 8, no. 1 (2015): 16. https://doi.org/10.3390/nu8010016.

5. Meng et al., "Roles of Chlorogenic Acid on Regulating Glucose and Lipids Metabolism: A Review," *Evidence-based Complementary and Alternative Medicine: eCAM* (2013): 801457. https://doi.org/10.1155/2013/801457.

6. Watanabe et al., "The Blood Pressure-Lowering Effect and Safety of Chlorogenic Acid from Green Coffee Bean Extract in Essential Hypertension," *Clinical and Experimental Hypertension* 28, no. 5 (2006): 439–449. https://doi.org/10.1080/10641960600798655.

7. Harpaz et al., "The Effect of Caffeine on Energy Balance," *Journal of Basic and Clinical Physiology and Pharmacology* 28, no. 1 (2017): 1-10. https://doi.org/10.1515/jbcpp-2016-0090.

8. Guest et al., "International Society of Sports Nutrition Position Stand: Caffeine and Exercise Performance," *Journal of the International Society of Sports Nutrition* 18, no. 1 (2021). https://doi.org/10.1186/s12970-020-00383-4.

9. Institute of Medicine (US) Committee on Military Nutrition Research, *Caffeine for the Sustainment of Mental Task Performance: Formulations for Military Operations* (Washington, D.C.: National Academies Press, 2001), 2. https://www.ncbi.nlm.nih.gov/books/NBK223808/.

10. Hoshimoto et al., "Caprylic Acid and Medium-Chain Triglycerides Inhibit IL-8 Gene Transcription in Caco-2 Cells: Comparison with the Potent Histone Deacetylase Inhibitor Trichostatin A," *British Journal of Pharmacology* 136, no. 2 (2002): 280–286. https://doi.org/10.1038/sj.bjp.0704719.

11. St-Pierre et al., "Plasma Ketone and Medium Chain Fatty Acid Response in Humans Consuming Different Medium Chain Triglycerides During a Metabolic Study Day," *Frontiers in Nutrition* 6 (2019): 46. https://doi.org/10.3389/fnut.2019.00046.

12. Vandenberghe et al., "Tricaprylin Alone Increases Plasma Ketone Response More Than Coconut Oil or Other Medium-Chain Triglycerides: An Acute Crossover Study in Healthy Adults," *Current Developments in Nutrition* 1, no. 4 (2017): e000257. https://doi.org/10.3945/cdn.116.000257.

13. Östman et al., "Vinegar Supplementation Lowers Glucose and Insulin Responses and Increases Satiety After a Bread Meal in Healthy Subjects," *European Journal of Clinical Nutrition* 59 (2005): 983–988. https://doi.org/10.1038/sj.ejcn.1602197.

14. Kondo et al., "Vinegar Intake Reduces Body Weight, Body Fat Mass, and Serum Triglyceride Levels in Obese Japanese Subjects," *Bioscience, Biotechnology, and Biochemistry* 73, no. 8 (2009): 1837–1843. https://doi.org/10.1271/bbb.90231.

15. Carol S. Johnston, Cindy M. Kim, and Amanda J. Buller, "Vinegar Improves Insulin Sensitivity to a High-Carbohydrate Meal in Subjects with Insulin Resistance or Type 2 Diabetes," *Diabetes Care* 27, no. 1 (2004): 281–282. https://doi.org/10.2337/diacare.27.1.281.

16. A. N. McLendon, J. Spivey, and C. B. Woodis, "African Mango (*Irvinga gabonensis*) Extract for Weight Loss: A Systematic Review," *Journal of Nutritional Thereapeutics* 2, no. 1 (2013): 53-58. http://lifescienceglobal.com/pms/index.php/jnt/article/view/927.

17. Joe Schwarcz, "The African Mango: Can Its Seeds Really Help You Lose Weight?" *McGill Office of Science and Society*, March 20, 2017, https://www.mcgill.ca/oss/article/health-nutrition-you-asked/african-mango-can-its-seeds-really-help-you-lose-weight.

18. Ngondi et al., "IGOB131, a Novel Seed Extract of the West African Plant *Irvingia Gabonensis*, Significantly Reduces Body Weight and Improves Metabolic Parameters in Overweight Humans in a Randomized Double-Blind Placebo Controlled Investigation," *Lipids in Health and Disease* 8, no. 7 (2009). https://doi.org/10.1186/1476-511X-8-7.

19. A. K. Sawicka, G. Renzi, and R. A. Olek, "The Bright and the Dark Sides of L-carnitine Supplementation: A Systematic Review," *Journal of the International Society of Sports Nutrition* 17, no. 1 (2020). https://doi.org/10.1186/s12970-020-00377-2.

20. N. Longo, M. Frigeni, and M. Pasquali, "Carnitine Transport and Fatty Acid Oxidation," *Biochimica et Biophysica Acta* 1863, no. 10 (2016): 2422–2435. https://doi.org/10.1016/j.bbamcr.2016.01.023.

21. Alison Steiber, Janos Kerner, and Charles L. Hoppel, "Carnitine: A Nutritional, Biosynthetic, and Functional Perspective," *Molecular Aspects of Medicine* 25, no. 5–6 (2004): 455–473. https://doi.org/10.1016/j.mam.2004.06.006.

22. Dulloo et al., "Efficacy of a Green Tea Extract Rich in Catechin Polyphenols and Caffeine in Increasing 24-H Energy Expenditure and Fat Oxidation in Humans," *American Journal of Clinical Nutrition* 70, no. 6 (1999): 1040–1045. https://doi.org/10.1093/ajcn/70.6.1040.

23. Maki et al., "Green Tea Catechin Consumption Enhances Exercise-Induced Abdominal Fat Loss in Overweight and Obese Adults," *Journal of Nutrition* 139, no. 2 (2009): 264–270. https://doi.org/10.3945/jn.108.098293.

24. M. P. Godard, B. A. Johnson, and S. R. Richmond, "Body Composition and Hormonal Adaptations Associated with Forskolin Consumption in Overweight and Obese Men," *Obesity Research* 13, no. 8 (2005): 1335–1343. https://doi.org/10.1038/oby.2005.162.

25. Sugita et al., "Daily Ingestion of Grains of Paradise (*Aframomum melegueta*) Extract Increases Whole-Body Energy Expenditure and Decreases Visceral Fat in Humans," *Journal of Nutritional Science and Vitaminology* 60, no. 1 (2014): 22–27. https://doi.org/10.3177/jnsv.60.22.

26. Sudeep et al., "*Aframomum melegueta* Seed Extract with Standardized Content of 6-Paradol Reduces Visceral Fat and Enhances Energy Expenditure in Overweight Adults—A Randomized Double-Blind, Placebo-Controlled Clinical Study," *Drug Design, Development and Therapy* 16 (October 2022): 3777–3791. https://doi.org/10.2147/DDDT.S367350.

27. Sugita et al., "Grains of Paradise (*Aframomum Melegueta*) Extract Activates Brown Adipose Tissue and Increases Whole-Body Energy Expenditure in Men." *British Journal of Nutrition* 110, no. 4 (2013): 733–738. https://doi.org/10.1017/S0007114512005715.

28. Onakpoya et al., "The Use of *Garcinia* Extract (Hydroxycitric Acid) as a Weight Loss Supplement: A Systematic Review and Meta-Analysis of Randomised Clinical Trials," *Journal of Obesity* (2011): 509038. https://doi.org/10.1155/2011/509038.

29. S. Basak, and A. K. Duttaroy, "Conjugated Linoleic Acid and Its Beneficial Effects in Obesity, Cardiovascular Disease, and Cancer," *Nutrients* 12, no. 7 (2020): 1913. https://doi.org/10.3390/nu12071913.

30. Rahman et al., "Effects of Conjugated Linoleic Acid on Serum Leptin Concentration, Body-Fat Accumulation, and β-oxidation of Fatty Acid in OLETF Rats," *Nutrition* 17, no. 5 (2001): 385–390. https://doi.org/10.1016/S0899-9007(00)00584-0.

31. Sakono et al., "Combined Effects of Dietary Conjugated Linoleic Acid and Sesamin Triacylglycerol and Ketone Body Production in Rat Liver," *Journal of Nutritional Science and Vitaminology* 48, no. 5 (2002): 405–409. https://doi.org/10.3177/jnsv.48.405.

32. A. J. Smeets and M. S. Westerterp-Plantenga, "The Acute Effects of a Lunch Containing Capsaicin on Energy and Substrate Utilisation, Hormones, and Satiety," *European Journal of Nutrition* 48 (2009): 229–234. https://doi.org/10.1007/s00394-009-0006-1.

33. John Lieurance, *Melatonin: Miracle Molecule* (Sarasota: Advanced Rejuvenation Publishing, 2020).

34. R. J. Reiter, Q. Ma, and R. Sharma, "Treatment of Ebola and Other Infectious Diseases: Melatonin 'Goes Viral'," *Melatonin Research* 3, no. 1 (March 2020): 43–57. https://doi.org/10.32794/mr11250047.

35. Faridzadeh et al., "The Role of Melatonin as an Adjuvant in the Treatment of COVID-19: A Systematic Review," *Heliyon* 8, no. 10 (2022): e10906. https://doi.org/10.1016/j.heliyon.2022.e10906.

36. Mubashshir et al. "Therapeutic Benefits of Melatonin against COVID-19," *Neuroimmunomodulation* 30, no. 1 (December 2023): 196–205. https://doi.org/10.1159/000531550.

37. Minich et al., "Is Melatonin the 'Next Vitamin D'?: A Review of Emerging Science, Clinical Uses, Safety, and Dietary Supplements," *Nutrients* 14, no. 19 (2022): 3934. https://doi.org/10.3390/nu14193934.

38. Avci et al., "Low-Level Laser (Light) Therapy (LLLT) in Skin: Stimulating, Healing, Restoring," *Seminars in Cutaneous Medical Surgery* 32, no. 1 (2013): 41–52. https://pmc.ncbi.nlm.nih.gov/articles/PMC4126803.

39. M. R. Hamblin, "Mechanisms and Mitochondrial Redox Signaling in Photobiomodulation," *Photochemistry and Photobiology* 94, no. 2 (2018): 199–212. https://doi.org/10.1111/php.12864.

40. "Red Light Therapy and Its Effects on Fat Cells," Aesthetic Bureau, accessed November 27, 2024, https://aestheticbureau.com.au/red-light-therapy-and-its-effects-on-fat-cells.

41. Caruso-Davis et al., "Efficacy of Low-Level Laser Therapy for Body Contouring and Spot Fat Reduction," *Obesity Surgery* 21 (2011): 722–729. https://doi.org/10.1007/s11695-010-0126-y.

42. Endocrine Society, "People with Brown Fat May Burn 15 Percent More Calories," news release, April 28, 2020, https://www.endocrine.org/news-and-advocacy/news-room/2020/people-with-brown-fat-may-burn-15-percent-more-calories.

43. Šrámek et al., "Human Physiological Responses to Immersion into Water of Different Temperatures," *European Journal of Applied Physiology* 81 (2000): 436–442. https://doi.org/10.1007/s004210050065.

44. "Norepinephrine," Cleveland Clinic Health Library, accessed November 27, 2024, https://my.clevelandclinic.org/health/articles/22610-norepinephrine-noradrenaline.

45. Imane Hachemi and Mueez U-Din, "Brown Adipose Tissue: Activation and Metabolism in Humans," *Endocrinology and Metabolism* 38, no. 2 (2023): 214–222. https://doi.org/10.3803/EnM.2023.1659.

46. Straat et al., "Cold-Induced Thermogenesis Shows a Diurnal Variation That Unfolds Differently in Males and Females," *Journal of Clinical Endocrinology & Metabolism* 107, no. 6 (June 2022): 1626–1635. https://doi.org/10.1210/clinem/dgac094.

47. Jones et al., "Pre-cooling for Endurance Exercise Performance in the Heat: A Systematic Review," *BMC Medicine* 10, no. 166 (2012). https://doi.org/10.1186/1741-7015-10-166.

48. Sarah Klein, "Should You Cold Plunge Before or After a Workout? Why Timing Matters," *Peleton* (blog), June 3, 2024, https://www.onepeloton.com/blog/cold-plunge-before-or-after-workout.

49. Vienna E. Brunt and Christopher T. Minson, "Heat Therapy: Mechanistic Underpinnings and Applications to Cardiovascular Health," *Journal of Applied Physiology* 130, no. 6 (2021): 1684–1704. https://doi.org/10.1152/japplphysiol.00141.2020.

50. Jem L. Cheng and Maureen J. MacDonald, "Effect of Heat Stress on Vascular Outcomes in Humans," *Journal of Applied Physiology* 126, no. 3 (2019): 771–781. https://doi.org/10.1152/japplphysiol.00682.2018.

51. Pope L. Moseley, "Heat Shock Proteins and Heat Adaptation of the Whole Organism," *Journal of Applied Physiology* 83, no. 5 (1997): 1413–1417, https://doi.org/10.1152/jappl.1997.83.5.1413.

52. Fennel et al., "Effect of Heat Stress on Heat Shock Protein Expression and Hypertrophy-Related Signaling in the Skeletal Muscle of Trained Individuals," *American Journal of Physiology-Regulatory, Integrative and Comparative Physiology* 325, no. 6 (2023): R735–R749. https://doi.org/10.1152/ajpregu.00031.2023.

53. Bouchama et al., "A Model of Exposure to Extreme Environmental Heat Uncovers the Human Transcriptome to Heat Stress," *Scientific Reports* 7, no. 9429 (2017). https://doi.org/10.1038/s41598-017-09819-5.

54. Kunutsor et al., "Inflammation, Sauna Bathing, and All-Cause Mortality in Middle-Aged and Older Finnish Men: A Cohort Study," *European Journal of Epidemiology* 37 (2022): 1225–1231. https://doi.org/10.1007/s10654-022-00926-w.

55. Laukkanen et al., "Sauna Bathing Is Associated with Reduced Cardiovascular Mortality and Improves Risk Prediction in Men and Women: A Prospective Cohort Study," *BMC Medicine* 16, no. 219 (2018). https://doi.org/10.1186/s12916-018-1198-0.

56. "The Science Behind Earthing," *Rowland Earthing*, accessed November 27, 2024, https://rowlandearthing.co.uk/pages/science.

57. James L. Oschman, "Can Electrons Act as Antioxidants? A Review and Commentary," *Journal of Alternative and Complementary Medicine* 13, no. 9 (2007): 955–967. https://doi.org/10.1089/acm.2007.7048.

58. Chevalier et al., "Earthing (Grounding) the Human Body Reduces Blood Viscosity—a Major Factor in Cardiovascular Disease," *Journal of Alternative and Complementary Medicine* 19, no. 22 (2013): 102–110. https://doi.org/10.1089/acm.2011.0820.

59. Howard K. Elkin and Angela Winter, "Grounding Patients with Hypertension Improves Blood Pressure: A Case History Series Study," *Alternative Therapies in Health and Medicine* 24, no. 6 (2018): 46–50. https://pubmed.ncbi.nlm.nih.gov/30982019.

60. Stephen T. Sinatra, "Grounding Q&A," *Heart MD Institute* (blog), last modified April 13, 2023, https://heartmdinstitute.com/q-a/grounding-q-a/.

61. S. O'Mara, *In Praise of Walking: A New Scientific Exploration* (New York: W. W. Norton & Company, 2020).

62. University of Massachusetts Amherst, "Meta-analysis of 15 Studies Reports New Findings on How Many Daily Walking Steps Needed for Longevity Benefit," *ScienceDaily*, March 3, 2022, https://www.sciencedaily.com/releases/2022/03/220303112207.htm.

63. European Society of Cardiology, "The More You Walk, the Lower Your Risk of Early Death, Even If You Walk Fewer Than 5,000 Steps," *ScienceDaily*, August 8, 2023, https://www.sciencedaily.com/releases/2023/08/230808201935.

64. National Heart, Lung, and Blood Institute (NHLBI), "Keep Walking: Study Finds Higher Daily Step Count Helps Adults Live Longer," news release, September 3, 2021, https://www.nhlbi.nih.gov/news/2021/keep-walking-study-finds-higher-daily-step-count-helps-adults-live-longer.

65. Bellini et al., "The Effects of Postprandial Walking on the Glucose Response after Meals with Different Characteristics," *Nutrients* 14, no. 5 (2022): 1080. https://doi.org/10.3390/nu14051080.

66. J. Inchauspé, *Glucose Revolution: The Life-Changing Power of Balancing Your Blood Sugar* (New York: Simon & Schuster, 2022).

67. Glucose Goddess. (n.d.). "Jessie's Research on Meal Pairing." Retrieved from glucosegoddess.com.

68. Inchauspé, J. (2021). "The Science of Blood Sugar and Metabolic Health." Journal of Nutritional Biochemistry.

69. Inchauspé, J. (2020). "The Impact of Meal Sequencing on Weight Management." Metabolism Clinical and Experimental.

70. Shukla et al., "Food Order Has a Significant Impact on Postprandial Glucose and Insulin Levels," *Diabetes Care* 38, no. 7 (2015): e98–e99. https://doi.org/10.2337/dc15-0429.

71. S. Imai, M. Fukui, and S. Kajiyama, "Effect of Eating Vegetables Before Carbohydrates on Glucose Excursions in Patients with Type 2 Diabetes," *Journal of Clinical Biochemistry and Nutrition* 54, no. 1 (2014): 7–11. https://doi.org/10.3164/jcbn.13-67.

72. Shukla et al., "Carbohydrate-Last Meal Pattern Lowers Postprandial Glucose and Insulin Excursions in Type 2 Diabetes," *BMJ Open Diabetes Research & Care* 5, no. 1 (2017): e000440. https://doi.org/10.1136/bmjdrc-2017-000440.

73. Kubota et al., "A Review of Recent Findings on Meal Sequence: An Attractive Dietary Approach to Prevention and Management of Type 2 Diabetes," *Nutrients* 12, no. 9 (2020): 2502. https://doi.org/10.3390/nu12092502.

Chapter 12

1. Price Pritchett, *You^2: A High Velocity Formula for Multiplying Your Personal Effectiveness in Quantum Leaps* (Dallas: Pritchett & Associates, 1994), 15.

2. Robert Waldinger and Marc Schulz, "What the Longest Study on Human Happiness Found Is the Key to a Good Life," *The Atlantic*, January 19, 2023, https://www.theatlantic.com/ideas/archive/2023/01/harvard-happiness-study-relationships/672753.

INDEX

ACKNOWLEDGMENTS

Writing a book is never a solitary journey. It begins with a spark of inspiration, and is nurtured by countless conversations, extensive research, and an unwavering desire to make a difference in a world that is suffering. When I first envisioned *Metabolic Freedom*, I had no clear road map, but I committed to the journey, trusting that creativity would follow commitment. Reflecting on this process, I realize how fortunate I am to have the support of some of the world's leading thinkers, who have helped shape the ideas presented in these pages.

First and foremost, I want to acknowledge the Keto Kampers around the globe who engage with my social media content. To the millions who have watched my videos and listened to my podcast, thank you for your questions and comments. I know many of you feel lost, hopeless, and overwhelmed in your journey to heal your bodies, and I am deeply grateful for the trust you've placed in me. I commend you for taking control of your health. Reading about your victories and successes brings me immense joy, and my team and I celebrate them often. You are living proof of the body's incredible ability to heal itself.

In 2018, I attended a seminar in Boca Raton, Florida, hosted by Dr. Daniel Pompa. I remember it vividly. Within the first hour of hearing Dr. Pompa speak, I learned more about the body's healing potential than I had in a decade of studying nutrition. It felt as though he had completely reshaped my understanding of health, turning everything I thought I knew upside down. I told myself, "I want to learn everything he knows, and I want him to teach me." As Don Miguel Ruiz says in *The Four Agreements*, "Be impeccable with your word." I truly believe in the power of language, and shortly after making this declaration, I was personally mentored by Dr. Pompa. I had the privilege of working alongside more than 50 brilliant doctors and health practitioners through The Health Centers of the Future Platinum program. I've shared the stage with Dr. Pompa many times, and he has honored me by calling me his "greatest student ever." Dr. Pompa has been a tremendous inspiration, and this book would not have been completed without his brilliant work.

To my amazing team, who work tirelessly alongside me to serve our community: If you want to go fast, go alone. If you want to go far, go together. You are the best team I could have dreamed of. Thank you for joining me in this mission—I am forever grateful. Alina, Jonathan, Becky, Andrea, Sofia, Jeremy, Ian, Kamran, Christy, and Ada, thank you for your dedication to making a dent in disease.

A huge shoutout to all the incredible colleagues and mentors who have helped me piece together the metabolic puzzle. It has been an honor learning from each of you. Your research, friendship, and mentorship have been invaluable in helping me transform the lives of millions. A special thanks to Dr. Mindy Pelz, Dr. Jason Fung, Megan Ramos, Cynthia Thurlow, Reed Davis, Sean Croxton, Dr. Ben Bikman, Mark Sisson, David Asarnow, Shawn Wells, JJ Virgin, Roy Cammarano, Warren Phillips, Dr. Cate Shanahan, Dr. Will Cole, Dave Asprey, Ben Greenfield, Dr John Lieurance, Dr. Eric Berg and Dr. Ken Berry—your influence is deeply woven into my work.

Finally, I want to express my deepest gratitude to my family and close friends. Your belief in me has been the oxygen to my soul. To my mom, Haddi: Your sacrifice to immigrate to the United States from the Middle East has given me a life of freedom and opportunity. You are the most caring, unselfish person I have ever met. Thank you for your tremendous love and support. To my future wife, Natassia: Sharing my life with you has been one of the greatest blessings. Your unwavering support and love mean everything to me. Thank you for attending countless lectures and always being by my side. To my close friends Ronald, Carla, Alex, and Paul: Thank you for believing in me. Through tough times and times of triumph, you have stood by me. I am blessed to have you all in my life.

ABOUT THE AUTHOR

Ben Azadi, FDN-P, is a four-time Amazon best-selling author, international keynote speaker, and metabolic health expert with over 17 years of experience helping thousands reclaim their health. A recognized leader in the alternative health field, Ben is a pioneer in the keto and fasting movement, teaching the principles of a keto lifestyle, fasting, detox, hormone balance, and overall metabolic function.

His popular YouTube channel, where he shares the latest science-backed tools and techniques for resetting metabolism, has garnered over 25 million views. Ben is also the host of the *Metabolic Freedom* podcast, a top 15 podcast with more than 12 million downloads and over 900 episodes. The podcast was honored as Keto Podcast of the Year (2022) by the Metabolic Health Summit.

Ben's work has been featured in major publications, such as *Forbes, LA Weekly, Disrupt Magazine, New York Times Magazine,* and *LA Entertainment Weekly.* He also appeared in the groundbreaking documentary *Biohack Yourself* on Amazon Prime.

To learn more about Ben Azadi and his work, visit **benazadi.com**.

We hope you enjoyed this Hay House book. If you'd like to receive our online catalog featuring additional information on Hay House books and products, or if you'd like to find out more about the Hay Foundation, please contact:

Hay House LLC, P.O. Box 5100, Carlsbad, CA 92018-5100
(760) 431-7695 or (800) 654-5126
www.hayhouse.com® • www.hayfoundation.org

———

Published in Australia by:
Hay House Australia Publishing Pty Ltd
18/36 Ralph St., Alexandria NSW 2015
Phone: +61 (02) 9669 4299
www.hayhouse.com.au

Published in the United Kingdom by:
Hay House UK Ltd
1st Floor, Crawford Corner,
91–93 Baker Street, London W1U 6QQ
Phone: +44 (0)20 3927 7290
www.hayhouse.co.uk

Published in India by:
Hay House Publishers (India) Pvt Ltd
Muskaan Complex, Plot No. 3,
B-2, Vasant Kunj, New Delhi 110 070
Phone: +91 11 41761620
www.hayhouse.co.in

———

Let Your Soul Grow

Experience life-changing transformation—one video
at a time—with guidance from the world's leading experts.

www.healyourlifeplus.com

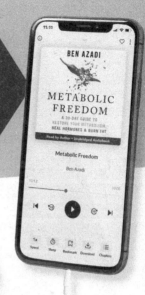